Intermittent Fasting
for Women

The Complete Beginners Guide for Weight Loss, Burn Fat, Learn to Heal your Body and Set a Healthy Lifestyle through the Self-Cleansing Process of Autophagy

professional before attempting any techniques outlined in this book.

By reading this document, the reader agrees that under no circumstances is the author responsible for any losses, direct or indirect, which are incurred as a result of the use of information contained within this document, including, but not limited to, — errors, omissions, or inaccuracies.

Table of Contents

Introduction

Congratulations on purchasing *Intermittent Fasting for Women* and thank you for doing so.

If you are an early bird, being most productive early in the day and usually in bed when the sun goes down, you can choose to eat earlier, say from 9am-5pm. For all the night owls out there, who see midnight on a regular basis, pushing you're eating window back to 4pm-12am is not problem at all. Any way you design your intermittent fasting plan is fine, so long as you follow the foundational rules: no calories during your fasting period (while still staying properly hydrated), and sticking to consuming all of your calories during the strict eating window that you designate.

If this is your first time of hearing intermittent fasting, you may be ready to close it immediately and never even consider this lifestyle. If that is you, this feeling is probably due to outdated fitness and nutrition advice that society and so-called "gurus" have hammered into your mind for decades. You have without a doubt heard that breakfast is the most important meal of the day, or eating 5-6 small meals every 2-3 hours throughout the day is the most effective way for efficient metabolism, or that 'starving' yourself in an attempt to lose weight is counterproductive, etc.

Before we even begin to debunk these myths with all of the benefits of intermittent fasting, you need to realize that this is not a new concept by any means. Eating throughout the course of the entire day is a relatively new concept. Food has become so convenient and accessible in today's society that we are trained into believing we need three square meals a day. Society is so concerned with eating, instant gratification of our dietary desires that there are fast food restaurants on every corner with their flashing neon signs advertising the latest $5 calorie bomb. Is it any surprise then, that obesity levels are soaring, heart disease and stroke are running rampant, and people are unhealthier than ever before?

From our earliest ancestors all the way up until a few hundred years ago, the habit of eating one large meal at the end the day was the norm. Ancient humans were hunter-gatherers, spending the entire day foraging for edible vegetation, hunting game, and just trying to survive. Eating was considered a celebratory ritual and was accompanied by a feast each evening when the food was brought back to the tribe. Even our modern ancestors spent their days farming the land, working whatever job needed to be done for their families, eating one large meal after a hard day's work.

While I am by no means saying that these people had it better than we do now (I would rather eat a few too many calories each day than have to survive a saber-toothed tiger attack), they did in fact reap many of the benefits of intermittent fasting without even realizing it. To digress, eating throughout the duration of the day is a relatively new concept that is not at all necessary to a healthy lifestyle.

Chapter : 1
Weight and Eating Problems in Women

We have discussed the science and effects fasting has on your body, but let's take that information and apply it directly to weight loss. We have mentioned weight loss regarding fasting, but how is this put into practice? You cannot simply fast for a week and expect drastic weight loss. However, by keeping fasting a part of our everyday diet, we allow our body to adapt to changes more easily, and thus can implement other practices that go hand in hand with fasting to ensure maximum results. Remember, weight loss is not only attributed to calorie restriction, but definable results are also seen with overall physical and mental health. Let's start with why we want to lose weight in the first place.

Physical appearance plays an integral role in our society. Billboards and commercials fill the air with super skinny models, forcing our minds to think that there is one true way women are supposed to look. This is completely unfair, and it attacks the mind as a whole. In good practice, we should try and avoid these thought patterns as much as possible and focus on our personal goals. Physically appearing attractive does not imply health. Too skinny, too fat – these words mean nothing if our bodies and minds are not balanced and healthy. So, let's find out why we want to cut weight with a few personal questions to ask ourselves: **Do I simply want to be beautiful? Do I want to lose weight for longevity? Is my body shape hindering me in some way? Do I need to lose weight for health purposes?** Even the healthiest of people will strive for more balance. No attainable end goal applies to everyone. You need to find your ideal goal and go from there. By taking time to contemplate why we want to or need to lose weight, we can hone in on our specific goals and aspire to attain them through specific practices directed at specific results.

Once we find ourselves being truthful with ourselves about body image, we can begin a true weight loss practice and with it a fasting regimen. But how will this fasting help us cut weight? Aside from the science showing us that Intermittent Fasting reduces inflammation, assists in hormone regulation, and burns cleaner energy, we need to view the fast through a psychological lens.

By even thinking about starting an IF routine, you have already started to change your life. The thoughts that cross your mind about wanting something better for yourself is just the beginning of what could become a dramatic life-altering transformation. The desire for longevity and to be healthful are very common goals; unfortunately, many people suppress these desires in exchange for an easier, way less healthy lifestyle. As this downward spiral progress, one becomes caught in a seemingly endless loop of processed foods, social media, and laziness. By digging ourselves out of the typical routine, we have the opportunity to reinvent ourselves, to break the wicked cycle, and begin a new life. IF is a great place to begin for this process – not only do you break the detrimental meal cycle, but you also begin to see changes in your thought processes about everything else in your life that may be preventing you from living a healthy and happy life. By being persistent and dedicated, we can begin breaking away from the standard lifestyle. By eliminating the unneeded stress, we also assist ourselves in losing our unneeded weight.

The relationship between stress and obesity has been studied extensively, and there is a link between the two. As the obesity rate began to increase quickly in the United States, scientists soon realized that the problem wasn't limited to only wealthy countries but was a global problem. Thought initially to be a product of overeating and lack of exercise, soon studies showed that many other factors contributed to this pressing issue. Obesity-related illnesses have been linked to industrial, cultural, and, of course, genetic predispositions –all being stressors that are out of our control. Our surroundings cause these stressors, and our society plays a huge role in weight management. Stress is a response in our bodies that is critical for survival. The 'flight or fight' response ensured our survival in prehistoric times and allowed us to adapt to our environment. When we are stressed, our autonomic nervous system is activated; this system regulates heart rate, blood pressure, hormone regulation, and digestion. As we see here, these are the same major functions that IF has been shown to help balance and regulate.

Many of the people who have problems with obesity react to stress by eating food. However, this 'comfort' food is not worth the trouble. Much of the comforting food is very high in fats and sugar, not to mention usually consumed outside of the individual's routine. This may serve as a quick fix for stress, but it can lead to addiction-like behavior and overeating. It is no secret that the food that is valued in our culture is not very healthy, and with the advent of GMO foods and soil that is depleted of nutrients from pesticides, even our fruits and vegetable are not up to par. The food problem is a huge issue today, in fact, unavoidable, but there are ways we go about our lives that counteract much of the problem. Eating nutrient-rich foods that are grown locally and avoiding frozen or prepackaged meals will go a long way to reduce stress. We will go into detail about the suitable meals for IF in a later chapter. By being mindful about our relationship with food is only going to help us in our journey to transformation.

Another issue with weight loss is physical activity. Many people feel that they do not have time to exercise or simply have become so out of shape that the idea of exercise never comes to mind: this is unacceptable. Some may hear the word exercise and instantly picture in their minds a sweaty, beefed-up man lifting weights in front of a mirror. This is a very narrow-minded approach to exercise. Instead of these stereotypical ideas of what it takes to be healthy, let's consider fewer intensive images. Someone in normal everyday clothing walking casually on a trail in the wilderness or perhaps slowly stretching on a yoga mat in a quiet room – this is exercise too. We don't have to hit the gym to have a balanced physical lifestyle, but simply moving around and getting the blood flowing can suffice. Studies have shown that stress is reduced with a casual exercise routine that even in the moments of the stressful situation, a quick stretch or walk around the block will help alleviate the stress. We will discuss the relationship between IF and exercise later.

So, we see that stress is an important aspect of weight management; it affects the very same major functions that IF has been shown to affect. Combined with a more mindful diet, moderate exercise, and truthful self-image, we see the formation of a very safe and effective routine for weight loss. Now, let's look at what is happening to excess fat when we are in the midst of a fast.

As discussed above, we have found that fasting improves health in many ways. The most accepted science on IF states that fasting influences the circadian rhythms and various other systems needed to live. Circadian rhythms are built in biological processes that act like a biological clock, similar to other natural rhythms such as the tides or seasonal rhythms. These rhythms are controlled by the hypothalamus and can be altered and trained from outside influences, such as light, darkness, food, and IF, respectfully. Organs in your body respond to food restriction and can act to reset these rhythms. Food restriction also affects the microbiome of your gut – all the bacteria and ecosystem of your gut has its own rhythm as well. As your body resets and the energy from your latest meal is used up, the body turns to fat reserves. The fat reserves release fatty acids which find their way to the liver where they are then converted into ketones. The ketones provide energy for muscles and help to prevent disease processes by protecting neurons. Although, if ketone levels become too high, it could be dangerous. This complicated process is the underlying physical benefit of IF: resetting the internal clocks and using fat reserves. The fat reserves having been reduced, we now find ourselves weighing less safely and effectively. When considering this, we need to dig a little deeper into what ketosis is and how it works.

Ketosis

Much information you find online about IF or weight loss leads to websites and articles dedicated to ketosis and keto diets. Although the ketosis diets are not mandatory for IF, it is a good idea to be educated on the process of ketosis itself and how it interplays with IF.

Ketosis pops up a lot in conversations about health and current diet trends; it is one of the more popular diets on the Internet and yields plenty of success stories from people who practice the diet. But what is ketosis exactly? It can be a positive or a negative thing depending on the context and situation. Ketosis is a natural process that occurs in the body as a metabolic process. Similar to what we've discussed, when your body doesn't have any quick energy to burn, such as carbohydrates from a recent meal, it will burn stored fat instead. This process makes ketones. If the ketone levels in the blood get too high, there can be complicated problems – typically insulin and other hormones prevent the ketone levels from getting too high. However, if there are issues with insulin production, this can be an issue. This is why people with diabetes find themselves in an unwanted ketosis state if they're not using enough insulin and often avoid inducing the state intentionally. A healthy normal body that consumes a balanced diet is in control of the amount of fat it burns and typically won't make ketones. Aside from just restricting carbohydrate intake, ketosis can also be induced by pregnancy and long exercise routines. The ketosis state can most certainly be viewed as a survival mechanism built into the human body. When we have no quick energy to use, or we have no food to ingest, our body switches over to creating ketones and using stored fat to power the body. We see here how ketosis fits into our IF lifestyle. If we restrict calories, especially from carbohydrate-rich foods, the ketosis state will take hold, and we can start burning unwanted and excess fat.

As a weight loss strategy, ketosis diets are effective and safe when practiced with attention to our bodies and state of mind. Not unlike a paleo diet or the popular Atkins diet from decades ago, the low-carb strategy can be very beneficial if used wisely. The diet has been shown to assist the body to maintain muscle and make you feel less hungry. Obviously, fasting will induce a ketosis-like state very quickly, but reducing carbohydrate intake to less than 60 grams a day for four to five days can start a ketosis-like state as well. The diet has been implemented to some success for treatment of many serious diseases including epilepsy.

As with any diet, a ketogenic diet needs to be practiced with great care and with meticulous attention to your body's changes. If the ketone levels in your body get too high, they can build up in the blood and ketoacidosis can take hold. Ketoacidosis causes the built-up ketones to turn the blood very acidic and can result in a coma or even death. Ketone levels can be tested in urine or blood, and it is always a good idea to test if you choose to practice a ketogenic diet. Along with unsafe fasting practices, ketoacidosis can be caused by alcoholism, dehydration, and an overactive thyroid. If you are affected by these symptoms, it is best to check with your doctor before attempting any diet or fast that may induce a ketogenic state.

So, not only do we see an IF routine as directly affecting our circadian rhythms and reducing fat, but the practice acts as a building block to other weight loss protocol. Through fasting, we influence the systems of the body that cause stress, while simultaneously taking societal stress off ourselves by developing a better diet and attitude. The IF routine affects our idea of exercise, not only by freeing time to exercise but also by inducing a ketosis-like state and exercising. We burn fat reserves quicker than if we were eating the same foods at the same time. This combination will be the basis of our weight loss regimen. Now, we need to find a fasting technique that is best suited to our needs.

As we continue on our transformative journey, with science in mind, we need to explore the many different ways we can introduce IF into our lives. There is an infinite number of ways to start your IF routine, but we will focus on some of the more prominent methods that have taken the Internet by storm in recent years.

Chapter : 2
Fasting

As the popularity of Intermittent Fasting grows, many voices can be heard speaking negatively about the practice. This is understandable as fasting is a taboo in the Western-developed world, seemingly depriving oneself of necessary nutrition would frighten anyone with a conscience. Fears pertaining to exercise are very common. It would seem that not having any food intake would make exercise out of the question, but it will depend on the type of exercise and, of course, your overall health. It is very important to read this section thoroughly, so you don't contradict the work you've done to better yourself. Many myths can be found online, but let's analyze these allegations and apply the science we've learned to debunk any fears and ensure the safest and most effective means of exercise while Intermittent Fasting.

We've seen the science of this kind of fasting allowing our body to use our fat reserves for a cleaner and more efficient energy, but is exercise going to disrupt this process? And if not, what exercises are the most useful? Here we will discuss an IF and exercise combination, while also debunking some other myths pertaining to exercising on an empty stomach.

Let's start with some basic misconceptions about fasting:

Intermittent Fasting Will Slow Your Metabolism

This is a very misunderstood concept. While you fast, your body is going to try to compensate for the disrupted meal routine, but your metabolic rate will not slow; it will simply go about its business as usual. If your body were somehow to use up all its energy and fat reserves, then you would be considered to be 'undereating', and this is when the metabolism slows, and you could be in potential harm's way. So, instead of focusing solely on the idea that fasting is calorie restriction, view it as more of a restriction of the time when you're allowed to intake calories.

By Just Fasting You Will Lose Weight

As we have discussed, losing weight isn't going to happen overnight just because you restrict calories. Developing a nutrient-rich diet alongside casual exercise with IF fasting will be much more effective. Eating pizza every chance you get is not a mindful approach to fasting or a balanced diet, which leads us to the next myth.

You Can Eat Anything You Want In Between Fasts

Ending a fast then diving into a processed food coma is about as counterproductive as it gets. Maintaining healthy eating habits outside of fasting days is going to be a very important key to losing weight and keeping it off. Try to avoid using your fasting practice as an excuse to overindulge.

Intermittent Fasting Is Effective and Everyone Sees Results

This has been a big one throughout the book. No one practice is going to suit everyone. Each individual is very different. Although we all share a basic structure, genes and environment play a huge role in what practices work and what doesn't. Let's not be discouraged though; we can customize our practice and find what works best with just a little time and effort.

Fasting Is Starving Yourself and Unhealthy

We've touched on this one, and it is very common. You express to a peer that you're going to start fasting and they are taken aback by your statement. They think you're going to get hurt or starve to death, and this just isn't true. We've discussed the science, and if used correctly, these ancient practices are safe. Let us keep in mind that we are transforming ourselves through fasting; we are using it as a structure and foundation to a healthy and happy life.

Fasting Leads to Muscle Loss

This is a popular argument for people who oppose fasting. However, the truth is that muscles that are used on a regular basis and plenty of protein ensure the muscle's health. In fact, if the body is searching for fuel, it is not likely to go after muscle since stored fat is way more efficient. Keep in mind, though, that you do not have unlimited fat reserves.

Now, for some myths regarding exercise in general, there is much debate among scientists and people all around the world about what counts as proper exercise and which workouts and regimens are the best. We will continue on our path of 'Everyone is individual and requires customized fitness' as we explore these common misconceptions.

Exercising Leads to Weight Loss

Yes, you need exercise to stay fit, but exercise alone will not suffice. Do not assume that if you eat a pizza, you can simply go 'run it off'. Most studies show that to lose weight, you need balanced eating habits and regular exercise. In fact, many agree that a balanced diet plays an even bigger role in weight loss than the exercise itself.

The Best Time to Exercise Is in the Morning

Exercising in the morning is a popular routine that many people adhere to, but this doesn't mean that it's the best time. Some studies show that exercise in the morning may help prime the body for fat burning during the day, but that's no reason to force a workout in the morning. The best time to exercise is when you feel is the best time. If you like late night runs, go for it. Do what you feel happy doing and make sure to keep active regularly.

Exercise Benefits Only the Physical

Another misconception is that the brain cannot be 'worked out' through exercise. This is untrue. Although puzzles and games help the brain, aerobic exercise seems to be the key to keeping your brain in shape.

Fasted Workouts

With these myths in mind, let's move on to some science about the combination of fasting and exercise or 'fasted workouts. These workouts are very popular for morning fasts since you can wake up with a relatively empty stomach, have some water, and hit your workout. However, there is much controversy on the subject of exercise on an empty stomach. There are not many studies available on the practice specifically, so the debate continues. Whether or not you think it works better than exercise on a half-full stomach or not, this book is here to give you suitable information to make your own informed decisions.

So, we know that when the stomach is empty, and the body has no immediate access to energy, then it will rely on stored fats. This fact alone implies that working out during a fast would successfully burn unneeded fat reserves, thus leading to weight loss. Although weight loss is the main focus here, we also need to address the many other benefits that IF has when combined with exercise. Studies have shown that fasted cycling to enhance endurance was easier to recover from than endurance cycling with food in the stomach. Along with recovery from endurance exercises, we have seen an improved recovery from the wear and tear of weight training, so we see a pattern of improved recovery after a workout if the athlete was in a fasted state. Similarly, fasted workouts should have higher glycogen storage. By keeping glycogen levels low during workouts, your body adapts to running on low glycogen. Thus, when you have food in your stomach, the body will use its energy more efficiently since it is trained to do so.

These ideas may not be the most amazing practices for a professional athlete, but for a regular person looking to shed a few pounds or develop a new lifestyle, the practices seem optimal.

But what about the many different types of exercise?

Most experts agree that exercise is safe to do while on an empty stomach, but are you getting the most out of your workout? As far as we can tell, the following conclusions can be found:

If your workout requires high levels of speed and power, you will benefit from having food in your stomach. This is due to the high amount of energy you will be burning in a short amount of time, so the energy that is available to be burned quickly is ideal for getting the most out of your workout.

For an empty stomach or fasted workout, the experts suggest cardio and aerobic workouts on all levels, whether it's tai chi or a jog through the park, or intensive yoga and deep stretching. These less intense workouts are ideal practices during a fast and will be the most effective for weight loss.

It is also understood that if you wish to start a fasted cardio routine, you should not have any serious health conditions like low blood pressure or other conditions that may cause dizziness or increase the risk of injury. The following tips are a great guideline for beginners:

1. Stay hydrated. Consume plenty of water.
2. Do not work out for longer than an hour
3. Choose moderate or low-intensity workouts
4. Listen to your body. If you experience discomfort, then take a breather

In the following chapters, we will reference 'light exercise'. This may be self-explanatory, but it will not hurt to suggest some exercise practices that pair well with IF. These exercises are light and not tough on the body, but we should still break a nice sweat when we are performing these 'light' exercises.

Some fitting ideas for fasted exercise:

- **Yoga**

Sanskrit for 'union', this traditional Indian practice sets out to unite the body and mind by combining intricate poses and stretches with structured breathing exercises. Cultural influence aside, even spending ten to fifteen minutes a day dedicated to stretching the body and focusing some attention on deep breathing will do wonders as a warmup to a workout or a workout in and of itself.

You can find plenty of books and online resources to find a yoga practice that suits you. The practice aims to strengthen the body while also furthering flexibility. It is a great core workout and really assists us in getting to know our body and its boundaries.

- **Tai Chi**

As a traditional Chinese martial art, this practice is designed to teach the practitioner how to control and manipulate the subtle energies of the body and its surroundings. Somewhat similar to yoga, this practice involves the constant movement of postures rather than holding poses. Breath is just as important during tai chi as in yoga. As a general rule, being in control of your breathing is a key component to a mindful and healthy life.

There is an abundant amount of material on tai chi online, and many major cities have multiple tai chi instructors and classes that meet in groups or one-on-one. Finding a class that takes place in a natural or relaxing setting is ideal.

- **Jogging**

All of us are familiar with jogging. The casual running exercise aims to build endurance and stamina by running at a steady pace at moderate speeds. Early morning jogs are a great way to start the day and pair well with a fasted morning.

You can jog anywhere. Jog around the block of your neighborhood or visit a school track or a gym that has running space to change the scenery. There are many running groups online if you feel uncomfortable running alone.

- **Cardio**

Cardio workouts are defined as any workout that gets your heart rate up. Jogging can be considered cardio, but there are meticulously designed cardio workouts that aim to burn fat through different intensities. Many workouts ask that you have intervals of intense cardio followed immediately by rest than more intense cardio.

There are hundreds of different cardio styles and workouts available online to suit your skill level and lifestyle. Your local gym should have machines perfect for cardio and possibly even classes dedicated to weight loss through cardio. Cycling machines and the elliptical are popular machines you can find at gyms for cardio workouts.

- **Pilates**

Very similar to yoga, but with more strength building exercises, Pilates was invented in the twentieth century as an effective way to tone muscle without bulking up. It pairs well with IF since it is low impact and can be performed anywhere, not unlike yoga.

Most cities should have Pilates instructors nearby, and there are abundant resources online.

- **Hiking**

This is a low-impact, relaxing, and thought-provoking activity. Taking a hike in the woods is an immersive experience. There's something very beneficial about being in a natural setting away from all the hustle and bustle of a town or city. Depending on the terrain, hiking can be a casual stroll or close to a treacherous climb. The combination of fasting and hiking is an amazing one as you notice your senses are heightened as you walk empty-bellied through the forest.

There are hiking trails all around the world, and they often state the intensity level of the hike. Searching for new trails and scenic spots quickly becomes a hobby that is beneficial on many levels. Adventurous, educational, self-reflective, and most certainly great for your body, hiking is paired wonderfully with IF since you are in control of how difficult it is. But, of course, if you are fasting and going out into the woods, be sure to bring plenty of water and emergency snacks.

Chapter : 3
Intermittent Fasting for Women

Advantages

Weight loss is probably the main reason why this diet is quite popular. Weight loss is a great benefit, but this diet offers more than just this. In this section, you will learn about the different benefits of this popular dieting protocol.

Lose Weight

The most popular and obvious benefit of intermittent fasting is weight loss. Intermittent fasting oscillates between eating and fasting periods. This obviously results in a reduction of your total calorie intake. Unless you go overboard and try to compensate for the fasting hours by binging too much when you break the fast. Fasting helps with weight loss as well as maintenance of the weight loss. Fasting is also a great way to prevent from indulging in mindless eating. As mentioned earlier, whenever you eat something, your body immediately converts it into glucose and fat. When you skip a meal or two, then your body starts to burn fats to meet the energy requirements. When your body reaches into its internal fat stores, it leads to weight loss. A significant portion of the fat cells is present in the abdominal region. So, if you want a flat tummy, then this is a great diet.

Better Sleep

One of the major health problems these days is obesity. In fact, obesity is a marker for various diseases and illnesses. Lack of sleep is a primary cause of obesity. Whenever your body is deprived of the rest it needs, then your internal mechanism of burning fats slows down. Intermittent fasting helps regulate your sleep cycle, and it also makes your body's fat burning mechanism effective and efficient. Good sleep has psychological benefits as well. Your energy levels will stay high when you get a good night's sleep.

Improves the Resistance to Illnesses

Intermittent fasting kickstarts autophagy. Autophagy helps with the regeneration and removal of damaged cells. This is a natural process, and intermittent fasting makes it more efficient. This helps to improve the overall functioning of your cellular components. When this happens, then your body is better equipped to deal with illnesses.

Improves Heart Health

Intermittent fasting helps with weight loss and this, in turn, helps improve the functioning of your cardiovascular system. The buildup of plaque is the leading cause of several cardiovascular diseases. The buildup of plaque is known as atherosclerosis, and in this condition, the thin lining of blood vessels (endothelium) don't function effectively. Obesity is one of the major reasons for the increase in plaque deposits. Stress or inflammation tends to worsen this situation even further. By tackling obesity, it directly helps reduce the risk factors associated with cardiovascular diseases and as a result, improves your heart's health.

Improves your Gut's Health

Are you aware that your gut is home to millions of microorganisms? The symbiotic microorganisms are known as microbiome assist the functioning of the digestive system. Intermittent fasting ensures that these microbiomes are functioning optimally and this, in turn, improves the gut's health and improves in better assimilation and absorption of the food you consume.

Managing Diabetes

Diabetes is quite troublesome by itself. It is a primary aggressor for cardiovascular dysfunction that leads to different health problems like heart attacks and strokes. Your body releases insulin whenever you consume food; however, when the level of glucose increases in the bloodstream, and there isn't sufficient insulin to deal with it, it causes diabetes. Diabetes also leads to your body developing resistance to insulin, and this makes it difficult for your body to manage insulin levels. Intermittent fasting helps decrease sensitivity to insulin and this, in turn, helps manage diabetes.

Reduces Inflammation

Your body's natural defense mechanism to deal with any internal problems is inflammation. Inflammation is helpful in moderation, and it helps fight off any foreign bodies; however, if left unchecked, inflammation can be quite troublesome. A high level of inflammation causes metabolic dysfunction and leads to different painful conditions like arthritis, atherosclerosis and other degenerative diseases. Such inflammation is known as chronic inflammation, and it is a rather painful condition. Intermittent fasting helps control chronic inflammation.

Promotes Cellular Repair

Intermittent fasting helps kickstart autophagy. Most of the diseases related to the aging of the brain take a long time to develop since the proteins present in and around the brain cells are misfiled, and they don't function like they are supposed to. Autophagy helps clean up all these malfunctioning proteins and reduces the accumulation of such proteins. For instance, in Alzheimer's, autophagy helps remove amyloid and α-synuclein in Parkinson's. In fact, there is a reason why it is believed that dementia and diabetes go hand in hand with each other — the constantly high levels of blood sugar prevent autophagy from kicking in and this makes it quite difficult for the body to get rid of any damaged or malfunctioning cells.

Methods and different Type of Intermittent Fasting?

Intermittent fasting is a very popular diet and has several variations. In this section, you will learn about the different variations of intermittent fasting that are ideal for women.

Crescendo Method

Intermittent fasting protocols are fairly simple, but it can be difficult for your body if you do not know much about fasting, start too fast or make any radical changes. So, if you're interested in starting with a pattern of intermittent fasting, it's better to start with the crescendo method. With this method, you have to fast for a few days a week instead of observing a daily fast. This is a rather mild approach to the intermittent fasting, giving you and your body a chance to get used to the new diet. It's a good idea to familiarize your body with the idea of fasting gradually. A radical all-or-nothing approach may sound good in theory; however, if you are getting used to this diet and want it to be sustainable in the long run, a slow start is a good idea. You can take full advantage of intermittent fasting without causing imbalances in your body. As mentioned in the previous chapter, a woman's body is very susceptible to changes in nutrient intake. So, if you are not careful, it can cause metabolic disorders and imbalances. To avoid this, it is a good idea to introduce your body to any change gradually.

By following the intermittent fasting protocols, you can lose all the extra pounds that have accumulated. You can use any other intermittent method described in this section; however, it is a good idea to start with this method before proceeding with any of the other post methods. The rules of a crescendo contribution are very simple and easy to follow, especially if you are unfamiliar with the idea of fasting.

According to the Crescendo Contribution protocols, you must fast for two or three days a week. Please make sure that you don't fast on two consecutive days. For instance, if you want to fast on Monday, then you must not fast on Tuesday too. Therefore, the ideal way to stay on this diet is to fast on Monday, Thursday, and Saturday. On fast days, make sure your exercise plan is nothing hectic. You can do less intense exercises like cardio or yoga. Please make sure that the duration of the fast does not exceed 12-16 hours. On other days, you can opt for any high-intensity exercises and eat as usual to give your body a chance to recover. You must always be sure that your body is constantly hydrated. So, you can drink any amount of no-calorie drinks. You can certainly fast for three days, but do not go beyond that.

16:8 Method

The 16: 8 method is also called the Lean gains method. This is an easy method of intermittent fasting that improves your body's ability to burn fat and improve muscle mass. This method requires you to fast for 16 hours daily. This means your food intake is limited to 8 hours on any given day. For instance, suppose you start fasting at 8:00 PM and keep fasting until noon the next day. Your first meal will be at noon and the last meal at 8 in the evening. So, your fast lasts for about 16 hours, and the food window lasts for 8 hours. If you start fasting on Monday night, then you will have to fast until noon on Tuesday. You can start with this fasting method as soon as your body gets used to fasting. This version of intermittent fasting is pretty simple. In fact, it can be as simple as skipping breakfast and having your first meal around noon.

Most people tend to skip breakfast, and if you're one of those people, you'll find that this method is very easy to follow. Yes, it is really that easy. After breakfast, enjoy a hearty and nutritious lunch, have a snack in the evening and finish the day with a healthy dinner. Once you have dinner, you must not eat anything until the next day. This method also helps to regulate your circadian rhythm. If you manage to eat your last meal by 8 pm, it means that your body has enough time to digest all of this food before you go to sleep.

The 24-Hours Fast

This intermittent fasting method is also referred to as the "eat, stop and eat" method. As the name implies, if you follow this variation of an intermittent fast, you must fast for 24-hours at a stretch. Note that you must not attempt to fast for more than two days a week. As mentioned earlier, you must not schedule fasting on consecutive days. You can select your fasting window, and if you opt for something then ensure that you stick to it as well. For instance, you can start your fast after dinner at 8:00 PM, and the fast ends at the same time on the following day. You can fast at any time, as long as it lasts for

24 hours. Whenever you fast, you can drink any calorie-free beverages. So, you can drink coffee, tea or whatever you like, if it contains no calories.

5:2 Diet

This diet is also referred to as a fast diet. According to the protocols of this diet, you have to fast two days a week. You may be wondering how this method differs from the crescendo protocol. If you follow this method, you can also eat on fasting days, provided you do not consume more than 500 calories. Two days a week, your calorie intake is 500 calories a day, and you can eat as usual on all other days. As already mentioned, don't plan your fast on consecutive days. It's up to you how you want to break calorie intake. You can eat one meal worth 500 calories or two small meals. It is up to you and your convenience.

There is another method of intermittent fasting that you can follow. This method has no clear structure and is quite simple to follow. You merely need to skip meals whenever you aren't hungry. Skipping a couple of meals now and then is fine. In fact, when you are caught up in work, it might happen that you don't feel like eating. In such situations, you merely need to skip a meal. That being said, there are a couple of things that you must keep in mind while you are fasting. You must never fast on two consecutive days. Ensure that your fasting period doesn't go beyond 24-hours. You must ensure that your body is thoroughly hydrated while fasting. Also, during the first couple of days, don't exceed 16 hours of fasting per day and never fast for more than three days a week. On all the days that you fast, your exercise schedule must be light and not intensive.

Selecting a Method

Now that you are familiar with the different methods of fasting, the benefits that come with it, and their potential drawbacks, you will need to choose a fasting method next. As you know, there are many options to choose from. How do you choose one of these methods? If you can answer the three simple questions that are covered in this chapter, you know your answer.

Before you choose a particular method, you need to know how important it is to choose a particular method of fasting. Why is it important to choose the right fasting method? You need to choose a method that suits you best, as it increases the chances of success of your diet. Choosing the ideal method not only increases the likelihood of dieting and reduces the likelihood that the diet will fail. If the option you choose suits your lifestyle well and you do not need to make an extra effort to follow it, you will probably stick to it. If you try to follow a fasting protocol that does not fit into your daily routine, it will only add stress. God knows that we all have sufficient things to worry about and we don't need another thing to worry about.

What Does your Normal Diet Look Like?

If your normal diet is high in processed foods, carbohydrates and sugars, fasting can be quite a difficult change. A diet rich in sugar and carbohydrates can be addictive to change, and if you choose a strict protocol, such as: As a dry fast or even a 16: 8 procedure, you will probably experience a few withdrawal symptoms. Once you experience symptoms of sugar or carbohydrate removal, it becomes difficult to follow a fasting plan. When this happens, you will most likely give up your diet prematurely.

Therefore, it is a good idea to start with the fasting protocol that recommends a fasting plan synchronized with your sleep plan. If you choose the 16: 8 method, most of your fast will be during sleep, and fasting will be easier. You can increase the duration of the fasting period gradually.

This is one of the main reasons why it is better to start fasting slowly. I mean, if you were to learn swimming, you will not dive into the deep end of the pool before you learn the basics, will you? If you are the "all or nothing," sort, then I recommend slowly getting used to the idea of fasting. You can start with gradual fasting, for instance, start with a 5: 2 diet before attempting strict fasting. You need to prepare your body and mind for fasting. If you are used to a sugar and carbohydrate-rich diet, gradually remove sugar and carbohydrates from your diet and replace them with healthier ones like protein and healthy fats. When you start removing unhealthy foods from your diet, the next step is to increase the time between meals gradually. If you are used to constantly preparing snacks, gradually reduce the number of snacks and increase the time between meals. Remember, it's about how your body is used to this diet. Work slowly with yourself, and you don't have to go cold turkey in the first attempt itself.

A radical approach will not benefit your body, and you must start slowly. You can take full advantage of intermittent fasting without causing harmful hormonal disturbances in the body. By following the protocols of this diet correctly, you can lose all the extra pounds you want. You can also use a different approach if you are not new to the post. The rules of this post are pretty simple. You have to fast two or three days a week, making sure you do not fast for days after. For example, you can fast on Tuesday, Thursday, and Saturday. On days when you are fasting, make sure the training protocol is simple, and you can do cardio or even yoga. Make sure that your contribution does not exceed 12-16 hours. On days when you do not want to fast and do not do high-intensity exercise, you usually need to eat to hold on to your energy. Keep your body hydrated, and you can even drink calories on hungry days. If you decide to fast two days a week, you can add another day in two weeks.

What is your Opinion about Fasting?

Fasting is both a physical and a psychological concept. So, ask yourself how comfortable you are with the idea of fasting. Do you agree with the idea of spending the whole day without food, or is it pleasant for you to fast a few hours? There are those who do not like the idea of fasting for an entire day, and they like short fasts. The best way to find this out is to test yourself. Try to fast for twenty hours (without food), and then dry fasting or even the 16: 8 method and it will be easy for you; however, if you have the idea of fasting where you are allowed to eat, select once a day or the option of fasting 5: 2.

I recommend that you pay attention to how you feel during the post. If you feel that this is fasting is a real struggle for you and you feel uncomfortable, you may not be able to stand up to strict fasts. So, stick with the shorter fasts initially. It all depends on your comfort. If you feel unwell, do not try to fast. If you want to make this diet sustainable for you in the long term, you must accept it.

What is your Daily Routine?

Fasting is pretty easy to follow even if you have a tight schedule. If you are busy with many other activities, such as your work, then you have no time to think about fasting or hunger pangs. If you are used to exercising in the morning, you have to choose a fasting mode that allows you to eat after exercise. Exercising will certainly increase your appetite, and you'll need to replenish your burnt calories to recover quickly. If you want to skip breakfast or do not like breakfast, you can choose the 16: 8 protocol.

Depending upon your lifestyle, personality and the goals you have set for yourself, the method of fasting can differ. Select a method of fasting that would easily fit into your life. If you are an early riser and you enjoy exercising in the morning, and you need to eat something in the morning after working out, you can adjust your feeding window accordingly. The eating window can be between 10 am to 4 pm. You can opt for the 24 hours fasting method if you don't want to fast daily. You can follow the warrior diet if you think you can get through the entire day with just one heavy meal at night. You will need to do plenty of research for figuring out the right diet for yourself. Go through the information provided in this book, check if your priorities and needs would fit in any of the methods mentioned.

As I said, you have to choose the method of fasting that suits you. If you find the fasting protocol difficult, do not forget that you have the option to customize it according to your schedule. This is probably the best part of the intermittent post. You will find one or the other that suits you, and you can easily follow that. Remember that with intermittent fasting, you do not have to give up on your lifestyle or diet to achieve your health and weight loss goals.

Disadvantages

In order to avoid these warning signs and to be able to continue without having to quit or recalibrate too intensely, glance over the following section of common mistakes. With the information at your fingertips, you should be able to avoid these pitfalls expertly and therefore succeed in your IF ventures. Whoever said it hurt to learn from others' mistakes? That's right, no one. Generally, the most common mistakes with intermittent fasting are as follows: eating incorrectly, stopping too eagerly, spending fast time incorrectly, or forcing things to happen.

Different situations/age in each woman?)

While the greatest concerns about intermittent fasting's effects on women often center on potential problems with reproduction and fertility, some women simply don't have to worry about that anymore. For mature and menopausal women, intermittent fasting poses a different instance and option entirely.

This chapter will be dedicated to the experiences of these women. It will discuss what happens when women age, how their needs change, and how nutrition is affected. Furthermore, it will discuss how intermittent fasting affects both mature and menopausal women before giving suggestions of how to approach IF for each type of woman.

Next, we will walk through some anti-aging foods, tips, and exercises to lose that weight, and then we'll end with the best intermittent fasting method for you at this time. By the time this chapter ends, you should feel confident (as a mature or menopausal woman) that you can approach intermittent fasting safely and productively, and you should have a solid plan in mind regarding how you'll go about that when you're ready.

Differences Between the Young vs. Older Woman

At the most basic level, it must be said that there are detailed bodily differences between young women and older women. Many of these bodily differences become obvious with the outward, physical effects of aging, but a lot of them also happen on the inside, away from what our eyes can see.

When women age, enter and exit menopause, and become fully mature, their bodies change, reflecting different nutritional needs for the next 30+ years. During menopause, in particular, certain foods help with the urges, hot flashes, and more, but the period of intense transition is more of a gateway into a completely altered future (mentally, bodily, nutritionally, and more).

Women of this age experience slowed metabolism (to their great frustrations) as well as lowered hormone production. For weight and mood, therefore, menopause and maturation are equal disasters. Your body will go completely "out of whack," compared to how it used to function. You'll likely put on weight despite the dietary choices you make, and you may feel there's no relief in sight. Don't be fooled, however! Things may have changed for you, but they won't be stagnant changes.

Essentially, women at the stage of menopause and beyond need to absorb less energy overall from their food, yet they need more protein to deal with the effects of aging. Vitamins B12 & D, calcium, and zinc will need to be boosted, while iron becomes less important for the aging female body. Vitamins

C, E, A, & beta-carotene need to be increased too in order to fight off cancer, infection, disease, and more.

As the woman ages and matures even further, more things will change; mainly, she cannot bypass taking these important supplements any longer. In older and more mature women, the body's abilities to recognize hunger and thirst become muted, and dehydration poses a greater threat. Fewer calories are required for the older and more mature woman too, but she still needs to get as many nutrients as (if not more than!) the young woman does.

It seems that a younger woman can eat (relatively) what she wants and not worry about taking vitamins or supplements, but it is undeniable that the older woman will need this nutritional help to ensure longevity. Basically, health needs become more pressing for women at this age, as their bodies are less flexible and resistant to problems that may arise.

How IF Affects Women at This Age & How to Approach It

Because health, diet, reproductivity, and nutritional needs are all altered for mature and menopausal women, their relationships with intermittent fasting can be very different from young women's. For instance, while young women ought to be careful about how intermittent fasting can affect their fertility levels, older women can practice intermittent fasting freely without these concerns. Therefore, more mature women can apply the weight-loss techniques of intermittent fasting to their lives (and waistlines) without worry of what negative side-effects might arise in the future.

For menopausal women, however, the situation is a little bit different than it is for fully mature women. People going through menopause have to deal with daily hormone fluctuations that cause hot and cold flashes, sleeplessness, anxiety, irregular periods, and more. At the beginning of this process, intermittent fasting *will not* necessarily help, and it could even make your situation more stressful.

For women in this situation who are actively going through menopause, you must remember that your body is extremely sensitive to changes right now. If you do find that intermittent fasting helps and that short periods of fast are effective, you *must* also make sure to increase the intensity of your fast as gradually as possible so your body can adjust without creating horrible hormonal repercussions for yourself and everyone around you.

For the fully mature woman, intermittent fasting will not make you as cranky, moody, irregular in the period, or otherwise because those hormones won't be affecting you at all anymore, or at least, hardly at all. Your dietary and eating schedule choices become more liberated from the effects they used to have on your hormonal health as the years go by. Therefore, if you're seeking weight loss, better energy, a physiological jolt back to health, or what have you, try out IF without concern and see what happens. For these types of women, intermittent fasting is set to provide hope through eased depression, the lessened likelihood of cancer (or its recurrence), promised weight loss, and more.

Anti-Aging Foods

Avocado is high in omega-3s, which help your immune system as well as your body as a whole fight inflammation.

Beans & Lentils are great sources of protein and fiber, particularly for older women.

Blueberries are high in vitamin C and antioxidants that help protect the skin from pollutants, sun exposure, aging stress, and more.

Broccoli, Cauliflower, & Brussel Sprouts are all relatively high in lutein which keeps your brain healthy and sharp!

Carrots are also rich in vitamin A as well as beta-carotene which helps your vision later in life.

Cilantro might taste like soap to some, but it helps remove metals from your body that shouldn't be there. It's a great detoxifier for women of any age.

Cooked Tomatoes have a powerful antioxidant present that helps the skin heal from the damage of any kind.

Dark Chocolate is packed with flavanols (which aid in the appearance of the skin and protect against the damage of the sun).

Edamame aids in bone health, cardiovascular healing, and ease into lowered estrogen levels with menopause.

Fortified Plant-Based Milk is a great non-dairy alternative to the "healing" animal milk you may know and love. They provide bone-supportive minerals and nutrients like calcium and vitamin D (as long as they're fortified!) without adding in the problematic nature of dairy to your healthy drink.

Ghee is a special form of clarified butter that is packed with healthy fats for skin health and detoxification.

Green Tea de-stresses the body and mind and blocks DNA from damage in many forms.

Manuka Honey is a special type of honey that's a powerful natural remedy for immune boost and skin health.

Mushrooms are high in vitamin D, which is so important for women of all ages.

Nuts are great at lowering cholesterol and fighting inflammation. They're also packed with fiber, protein, and micronutrients.

Oatmeal provides carbohydrates that encourage the release of serotonin, which keeps you feeling good.

Olives provide polyphenols and other essential phytonutrients that keep your DNA protected and your skin and body feeling and looking young.

Oranges, Lemons, & Limes, when juiced, provide the greatest source of healthy vitamin C you can imagine.

Papaya has many antioxidants, vitamins, and minerals that keep the skin elastic with fewer wrinkle lines.

Pineapples help maintain skin health, elasticity, and strength as you age.

Pomegranate Seeds are also high in antioxidants, and they're great at fighting free radical molecules that encourage the effects of aging on the body.

Red & Orange Bell Peppers have antioxidants and high vitamin C to help the skin retain its healthy shine while protecting it against pollutants and toxins.

Red Wine, when drunk in moderation, is a powerful tool to keep your heart healthy, lower cholesterol, and maintain muscle mass.

Saffron has anti-tumor, antioxidant, and other highly nutritious effects for the body.

Sesame Seeds will help you feel good through their high levels of calcium, magnesium, fiber, phosphorous, and iron.

Spinach & Other Leafy Greens work to protect the skin from sun damage while providing beta-carotene and lutein to solidify that effect.

Sweet Potato has more vitamin A than regular potatoes, which keeps your skin fresh and young-looking without lines and wrinkles.

Turmeric is great for the skin and for keeping the organs working in tip-top shape. The pigment curcumin also helps to heal DNA and prevent degenerative diseases.

Watercress is a happily hydrating green that's high in phosphorous, manganese, calcium, potassium, vitamins A, C, K, B1, and B2.

Watermelon works like a natural sun blocker when eaten and provides a great source of water to keep you hydrated.

Yogurt helps your cells stay young and is often probiotic, which is great for healthy gut flora and mood stabilization.

Chapter : 4
Self-Cleansing Process of Autophagy

Autophagy is when cells are able to clean themselves. It involves the process of a cell removing the toxins and other unwanted substances that might have penetrated their makeup. This would need to be done when a virus, bad bacteria, or other toxin has made its way into the body, regardless of the type of intruder versus cell attacked (Murrell, 2018).

Whenever a foreign particle might be present, then your cells will be able to fight that or remove it using autophagy. Autophagy occurs throughout the day without us having any idea what's happening. Your body is smart, so just because you're adding things to it that are damaging doesn't mean that it's always going to feel those effects.

Our bodies aren't perfect, however, so they will still need some help through other processes that can kickstart or encourage autophagy.

Cleaning of Waste Cells and Pathogens

The stronger the cell, the better it will be able to clean waste and get rid of various pathogens in the body. Fasting is a great way to encourage autophagy and cause your cells to not only rid themselves of toxins but to repair new, stronger ones as well (Murrell, 2018).

You might notice some detoxes are doing things aimed at specific detoxification, such as a liver detox, a heart detox, or even a brain detox. This isn't necessary, as encouraging autophagy throughout your body will help work to clean it starting from the inside, and eventually spreading all throughout your body.

Stop Progression of Diseases

Autophagy could even help encourage the reduction of cancer cells, or at least help to prevent them from growing in the first place (Bhutia, 2013). We have various mitochondria throughout our bodies that get older with time. Once they get to a certain age, they will start to release free radicals in our body. These could end up causing mutations, sometimes cancerous.

In order to produce new mitochondria and rid ourselves of the old, then we will need to focus on encouraging autophagy within our bodies. Caloric restriction is the best way to reduce this at first. This isn't a cure-all, but caloric restriction has been helped to slow down the production and growth of various tumors (Murrell, 2018).

This can be very specific, so it's important that you don't assume fasting is going to cure cancer. It might help prevent and reduce, but it's not necessarily a cure-all. In order to prevent it in the first place, encourage autophagy within your own cells.

How Autophagy Impacts You

Autophagy will have many other benefits to your health that are important to understand. It helps with reducing the amount of stored fat, which is a benefit in itself while also helping to prevent other health conditions associated with being overweight.

It can help repair damaged cells, which is important in order to keep up productivity from where those cells are damaged. For example, if some cells in your stomach are damaged from a life of unhealthy eating, autophagy could help to repair those.

All of this will also help reduce inflammation, which can have other serious health risks as well. When you experience inflammation, it can slow down certain processes and cause your organs to not work as well, depending on where the inflammation is present. When you get a cut, it turns red and swells – this is inflammation. When we damage our bodies inside, they will become inflamed; we won't see it.

This could have negative health effects, such as sore and tight joints, slow-working systems (such as a digestive system that isn't working properly/causes pain to use) and could even cause depression through an inflamed brain (Raison, 2011).

If you don't have autophagy within your body's function, it puts you at risk for some cardiovascular, rheumatological, atherosclerosis, and pulmonary diseases. You might also be at a higher risk of cancer, holding onto more fat, muscle loss, and even sensitivity to the sun.

Protein Cycling

One way to induce autophagy is to use protein cycling. This is the process of having some higher amounts of protein during some phases and lower at others.

When fasting, it will be best to reduce your protein intake on the days that you are restricting your food. On your days of eating and no fasting, then you can go back to a normal amount of protein. Fasting days stick to 25 grams or less. Other days, you can go back to normal, which is 46-56 grams depending on your sex/body weight.

The point of keeping yourself from eating too much protein will be to force your body to look elsewhere for its energy source.

When Autophagy and Protein Cycling Matter Especially for Women

These processes are important to include even in those that don't want to lose weight because autophagy will reduce overtime and become less efficient as we get older. This is especially important for women because we are at risk for certain estrogen-related diseases and cancers, and we usually have a higher fat content than the average healthy man. We want autophagy to work for us, and to reduce our body's toxins continually, so ensure that you are regulating your autophagy effectiveness through intermittent fasting.

How Autophagy is Related to Intermittent Fasting

We already know by now that fasting will make your cells turn on themselves, fat being burned along the process. Autophagy is your body's natural way of doing this, so it's clear to see that incorporating fasting will help to kickstart that natural process that already exists.

Autophagy occurs within the first 24 hours of fasting, on average. This means that you aren't fasting for 24-hours, but you've restricted your caloric intake. We will go over the actual methods of fasting in the next chapter so you can see what a 24-hour period might look like.

How to Induce Autophagy Through Intermittent Fasting

You might see supplements, teas, or other products that claim they induce autophagy, but the only clear way that's proven to be safe and effective is to do it naturally through fasting. As you fast, you are lowering your insulin levels. Therefore, you have a higher chance of starting autophagy within your body.

What's most important to induce autophagy is focusing on lowering your glycogen levels, which only shows after around 14 hours of fasting. For long health, you will want to include long periods of fasting for weeks, but preferably, months, at a time.

Chapter : 5
Keto diet

Our body is designed so that it receives the main energy for its work from carbohydrates – glucose. But this is "dirty fuel"; when it is "burned," many free radicals are released, which attack cells, damaging them. Another alternative way of obtaining energy is the splitting of fats, or more precisely the so-called ketone bodies. This is a cleaner option, which results in fewer free radicals being released, which means that the cells are less traumatized. Ketones begin to be used only in the case of a decrease in blood glucose. Therefore, in order to start a similar energy exchange, the amount of carbohydrates in the diet is reduced to a minimum, and the amount of healthy fats rises to a maximum.

Features of the diet

Let's face it, the diet is very "confused." Moreover, in order to achieve a result, it is necessary to strictly follow all the instructions. At the stage of entering the keto diet, in the diet there should be about 80% healthy fats, 10% protein, and 10% carbohydrates.

Healthy fats include nuts, seeds, olive oil and avocado oil, ghee, coconut fat, cream, avocado, small fish, organic lard (grown without hormones and antibiotics).

Carbohydrates: greens and leafy vegetables, cucumbers, zucchini, berries growing on the bushes: raspberries, blueberries, gooseberries, currants in small quantities.

Proteins: nuts, seeds, fish.

As you can see, the set of products allowed for consumption is not too wide. Yes, and with the transition to this type of power is associated with many difficulties. The first week of sitting on this diet is concerned with the so-called ketosis flu. The temperature may rise, chills or fever may appear. At this time, you need to drink more water, vitamins and be under the constant supervision of a doctor to control the transition period. By the way, at first, you need to constantly, about 3-5 times a day, measure the level of ketones and glucose in the blood. There are special test strips for measuring the level of ketones and glucose in the blood. This should be done to adjust the diet.

Who can use the keto diet?

As we already wrote, first of all, this diet is suitable for people with certain diseases, for example, diseases of the nervous system associated with the destruction of nerve cells. It is suitable for people suffering from Parkinson's disease, Alzheimer's disease, multiple sclerosis, diabetes mellitus, some autoimmune diseases. For the most part, these ailments bother people at any age, so be sure to talk about your ketogenic diet with your mother or grandmother. And such a diet can be recommended for cancer patients. A well-known fact: cancer cells can only feed on glucose and nothing else. Practically excluding carbohydrates from the diet, they are put on a rigid diet.

The benefits of the keto diet

On the ketogenic diet, general well-being and emotional mood are improved, a sea of energy appears, the brain begins to work at the speed of light, the ability to work increases, the concentration of attention increases. And with the help of such nutrition, you can negate the pathological dependence on sweet food. A large amount of fat in the diet allows you to achieve a feeling of fullness in a short time and for a long time. So, the thought of recharging with a bun or a chocolate bar is unlikely to come to anyone's mind.

What you should pay attention to

The ketogenic diet relates more to a healthy diet. There are a lot of pitfalls in it, so it is worthwhile going on this diet only for medical reasons and strictly under medical supervision. It is impossible, after reading about the wonderful bonuses of this diet on the Internet, to try to bring this type of food to life. Even with absolute health, it is possible to sufficiently undermine this very health.

Cons of this diet

If you decide to go on this diet, you should get acquainted not only with the advantages but also with the disadvantages of this diet.

A few days on the ketogenic diet can really lose weight. But the number of side effects like constipation, nausea, vomiting, kidney stones and changes in blood lipids make this diet just dangerous to health. "A sharp restriction of carbohydrates (glucose) in the diet leads to a state of hypoglycemia and to a periodic change of mood. A significant decrease in fiber intake in the body (vegetables and fruits), necessary for normal microflora, causes disruption of the gastrointestinal tract," explains Oksana Lishchenko. There may also be an unpleasant smell of acetone from the body, urine, and mouth due to a sharp increase in the content of ketone bodies in the body. On the one hand, it is a sign of attaining ketosis in the body, on the other hand, it is a reason to increase the amount of fluid consumed in order to get rid of this smell."

Due to the specific selection of products, there is no need to sharply limit the caloric intake for weight loss. Therefore, if you like fatty foods (meat, fish, avocados, nuts), then on this diet you will feel more comfortable than, for example, with a balanced but low-calorie diet.

Ketogenic diet. Composition and instruction

The basis of the ketogenic diet is a limited amount of carbohydrates, a moderate amount of protein, and fat as the main source of calories. Thanks to this food composition, after adaptation you will be stable in ketosis (read about it in our dictionary). The energy value of food on a keto diet looks like this:

Ketogenic diet calories composition

Fats are a source of 70-90% of calories on keto-diet

Here we look at the instructions with two ways to navigate in carbohydrates, proteins, and fats. The first is written for those who are not yet ready to meticulously count carbohydrates and calories. The second is for those who want to do everything "according to science".

I'll immediately warn readers who don't want "according to science": people have a poor understanding of the nutritional value of food in their mind. You may accidentally go on the wrong diet (the simplest thing is to overdo it with protein) and not see the result. Do not make hasty conclusions without trying the diet to the fullest extent.

To calculate the energy and nutritional values of your dishes, the best way is to use any application in your smartphone. There are a lot of them now, and some even suggest putting up a ketogenic diet as a goal.

From free calculators, I can recommend Fat Secret, suitable for Android and iOS. It is very popular and calculates the composition of calories, which is important for the ketogenic diet. It is in Russian. But I cannot vouch for it, as I myself use the cronometer.com service (the counter on the site is free, the application on the smartphone is paid). It is very convenient, but it is in English and there are no Russian products to choose from.

How many carbohydrates do you need to eat?

Carbohydrates here refers to digestible carbohydrates, that is, without regard to dietary fiber. Fibers are also carbohydrates, but they are not digested and do not affect the level of glucose in the blood. On food labels in Russia, they usually do not write what proportion of carbohydrates are fibers, so you can either assume that they are not there, or, if the product is typical, search the Internet.

The way "I want to try it"

Eat plenty of meat, eggs, green vegetables, oils, one handful of nuts or berries, and some fatty dairy products. So, you are unlikely to gain more than 20-30 grams of carbohydrates per day. But try not to overeat white meat, especially chicken or turkey. They have too much protein and little fat.

The way "I started; I will not stop there"

Use products from the list of low-carb, and count the number of carbohydrates per day, depending on your chosen level of severity of the diet:

Normal low-carb diet: 50-100 grams of carbohydrates per day. In this version, the diet may not even be completely ketogenic, that is, you will not be constantly in a state of ketosis. Because of this, you may feel weak (be sure to read about the ominous valley), but if this range is comfortable for you, do it.

Moderate ketogenic diet: 20-50 grams of carbohydrates per day. All the charms of the ketogenic diet with the ability to eat a few more nuts, berries, vegetables with starch or something else.

Strong ketogenic diet: not more than 20 grams of carbohydrates per day. Such a restriction is the standard of the ketogenic diet. It is in this performance that it is prescribed to people for therapeutic purposes: for epilepsy or cancer. But it is easier than it may seem.

Does it seem 50 or, moreover, 20 grams of carbohydrates is too little? So, it really can seem to an untrained person. After all, if we think of standard categories like "bread" or "porridge", then it will look like this:

In fact, in meat, fish, eggs, many vegetables and, of course, in oils, there are so few carbohydrates that you can eat them without even approaching the carbohydrate "ceiling".

Do not be afraid. Even on a strict ketogenic diet, one can eat variously and completely.

How much protein can you eat?

The amount of protein should be limited because the body has the ability to convert protein into glucose through the process of gluconeogenesis. And excess glucose can bring out the state of ketosis.

The way "Oh, let's just without formulas"

Eat 1.0-1.5 grams of protein for every kilogram of your weight. If you have significant excess weight, reduce the resulting figure by a third or divide in half.

The way "Hmm ... let's better with the formulas"

Approximately, the amount of protein should be around 1.0-2.5 grams per kilogram of your "fat-free" weight (about this below). The lower limit (1 gram) is in the case of a strict diet, and the upper limit (2.5 grams) in the case of a looser keto diet and during active sports.

To calculate the amount of protein you need, do the following:

Find out your weight.

To do this, use the usual weights. If you have scales that measure the percentage of body fat, this will help you with the next step.

Find out what percentage your weight is of fat.

You can use bioimpedance analysis tools built into household scales or sold as a separate device (for example, Omron meters). Passing a current through the body, they calculate the approximate proportion of fat through its electrical resistance. This is the most convenient, although not very accurate way. Other methods include measuring body fat with an instrument, ultrasound, and X-ray densitometry, which is considered the most accurate. We will not dwell on them here, as these are separate and extensive topics for discussion.

If you do not have analysis tools, you can estimate your percentage of fat per eye. This is not so difficult, especially since you do not need 100% accuracy – a rough estimate is usually sufficient. Look at photos on the Internet (just be careful!), Or use the following table:

Body fat percentage

Typical percentage of body fat in men and women (American Council on Exercise)

Accordingly, if you do not have excess weight, but the press dice is also not visible, then you can assume that it is about 25% fat for women, and 20% for men.

Further.

Calculate your "fat-free" weight using the formula = (your weight) × (1 -% fat)

Calculate the amount of protein you need by multiplying the calculated weight by the selected amount of protein from the range of 1-2.5 g / kg. Done!

Example. For a woman weighing 70 kg and 30% fat (0.3), who started going to a fitness club, the estimated amount of protein would be as follows:

Fat-free weight = (70 kg) × (1 - 0.3) = 70 × 0.7 = 49 kg

The amount of protein = (estimated weight) × (1.5 grams) = 49 × 1.5 = 74 grams.

Is it a lot or a little? So much protein is in two chicken breasts, 14 medium-sized eggs, or 10 ounces of a fat T-Bone steak.

How much fat do you need to eat?

In the ketogenic diet, fats are used as the main source of calories. And you should add them to carbohydrates and proteins that are already limited.

The way "what am I going to go with a calculator everywhere?"

If you eat the food in the list of products, then you are keto, and most likely 70% of your calories come from fat. Maybe even more. Well, it is, provided that the basis of your table are vegetables, fatty meat, fish and oils, and not berries.

And to go on a strict ketogenic diet, you will still have to count.

The way "Okay, I will go everywhere with a calculator"

After choosing the severity of our diet in terms of carbohydrates and proteins, you need to decide on the total caloric content.

You can use any calorie calculator online or use the following formula: 35 kcal per kilogram of your weight if you are not going to lose weight, or 30 kcal per kilogram for weight loss.

After you figure out how many calories you need per day, you can calculate how much fat you need to eat! It's very simple because we already know how many calories are derived from proteins and carbohydrates.

The example is already familiar to us. Suppose Marry wants to lose some weight.

Its weight is 70 kg. So, the amount of energy it needs is no more than $70 \times 30 = 2100$ kcal per day.

Marry chose a moderate diet with 30 grams of carbohydrates. Since 1 gram of carbohydrate gives 4 kcal of energy, of which it receives $30 \times 4 = 120$ kcal.

We have already counted the amount of proteins higher, and we got 74 grams. 1 gram of protein also gives 4 kcal of energy, so that Marry will receive $74 \times 4 = 296$ kcal.

It remains to get $2100 - 120 - 296 = 1684$ kcal! This is where we need fats. Since 1 gram of fat gives 9 kcal, the required amount of fat is calculated as $1684 \div 9 = 187$ grams.

Now we have all the raw data for Marry! To lose weight on a keto diet, she needs to eat 30 grams of carbohydrates, 74 grams of protein, and 187 grams of fat!

And what if Marry wants to maintain weight? Then recalculate her need for daily calories. She needs 70 × 35 = 2450 kcal per day. Then, without changing the number of proteins and carbohydrates, we calculate the amount of fat: (2450 - 120 - 296) ÷ 9 = 2034 ÷ 9 = 226 grams.

Making a menu on Keto Diet

For the standard version of Keto Diet

Calculate your daily calorie intake:

Add 500 kcal to build muscle

for fat burning - subtract 500 kcal from the number obtained

gram per 1 kg of dry muscle mass * kcal per 1 g

proteins 2.2 g 4 kcal

fats ** 1.8-1.88 g 9 kcal

carbohydrates 0,22 - 0,44 g 4 kcal

* Dry muscle mass is determined by the percentage of body fat. If you cannot measure it accurately, you can navigate through the picture.

** Fats are calculated last. After calculating the daily amount of calories for proteins and carbohydrates, the remaining number goes to fats.

Example

A man with a weight of 80 kg, height 175 cm.

The percentage of body fat - 20% (lean muscle mass - 64 kg).

The goal is fat burning.

Daily calorie intake is 2500 kcal.

For fat burning - 2500-500 = 2000 kcal per day.

Of them:

protein 2.2 * 64 = 140g (560 kcal)

carbohydrates 0,44 * 64 = 28g (112 kcal)

fat 2000-560-112 = 1328 kcal (150 g)

The easiest way to divide the calculated amount of proteins, fats, and carbohydrates equally into 4-5 meals. But this is not necessary, you can do each meal as you prefer. The most important thing is that the balance by the end of the day is in accordance with the calculations.

If you stick to the cyclic or targeted version of the Keto Diet, then on different days of the week the total caloric intake (due to carbohydrates) may differ.

Targeted Keto Diet

Add 0.5-1g of carbohydrate per kg of body weight before exercise. The point is to use all carbohydrates as fuel to increase the intensity of training. Fats should be reduced to the total caloric content to remained unchanged (for fat loss). You can divide the carbohydrates into 2 parts and one to use before training, and the second, after.

Cyclic Keto Diet

After the start of ketosis, about 2 weeks after the start of the diet (and then once a week), add 5-10 g of carbohydrates per 1 kg of dry weight per day. Such carbohydrate loading lasts from 9 to 36 hours. Start with 9, and then add 2-4 hours each time and evaluate the results. Please note that the amount of protein on such days remains high, and the fats need to be reduced. If you are on a fat burning diet, then in the days of carbohydrate loading calories can be raised to the level of the daily norm.

Is it possible to eat in the restaurant and at the same time not break the diet?

Keto diets are not only tasty and effective but also comfortable, as they require neither special products and methods of their preparation nor rejection of family and friendly lunches and dinners both at home and outside.

Here are three rules of going to a restaurant for those who want to enjoy food and socializing and not break the keto-diet.

1   You should see the menu in advance.

Friends called in a new place for you? Go to the site of the restaurant and explore the menu. And you will not pass for your companions as a bore and won't spoil the evening for yourself, for them, or even for the waiter and the cooks. I assure you, if you are not invited to any special set or to an institution that specializes in, say, cereals and fruits, you will certainly find at least three dishes that will suit you perfectly.

Keto restaurants – by analogy with vegetarian and vegan – are not yet available, but in the recently opened, keto-dishes are almost as common as ordinary ones. Tuna steak with avocado, tomatoes, and cilantro, and so on.

2   Adapt the dish according to the requirements of the keto diet

Did you find keto dishes in the restaurant menu that are extremely unlikely? Then look for options that could be easily adapted. How exactly? It is clear that it is not as in that joke: "I cooked everything according to the recipe, only instead of fish I took chicken, instead of parmesan — cheese, instead of mushrooms — oranges ... It turned out to be inedible in general, even the cat did not eat ...".

What is a hot meal in most cases? A serving of meat or fish plus a side dish - potatoes, rice, quinoa. Give up the side dish. Or ask for vegetables, and better with a low glycemic index: green salad, cauliflower or white cabbage, broccoli, asparagus, spinach. There are so many options.

Note: IF YOU KNOW THAT YOU ARE GOING TO THE RESTAURANT IN THE EVENING, REDUCE THE PORTION OF VEGETABLES AT BREAKFAST AND LUNCH. DO NOT EXCEED THE TOTAL NUMBER OF CARBOHYDRATES.

But it is even easier to increase the fat content in the dish – just ask the waiter to bring olive or butter (if they, of course, are no longer on the table). However, it should be borne in mind that you need only high-quality, "healthy" fats. So, it is better to ask whether the kitchen uses oils such as sunflower, corn, rapeseed, soy, etc.

3 You should remember the hidden sugar.

Sugar will break the keto diet and bring your body out of ketosis right away. Therefore, make sure that you do not accidentally fall into the hidden sugar, which can be contained in complex sauces, dressings, etc. If in doubt, for example, in a salad dressing, ask not to fill your salad at all, but to bring oil and vinegar separately. It is clear that it is unrealistic to prepare in advance for everything and it is still necessary to strain the waiter a little, but do it politely and carefully, and tell your friends that you care about their health because they don't need extra sugar either.

Differences between Keto Diet and Intermittent Fasting

Of course, everyone should watch out for their nutrition and not overeat. This is undoubtedly good for health. Many of us periodically notice that after a dense meal we become lethargic, drowsiness appears, the ability to work decreases, and we don't want anything except to lie down. All this testifies to the fact that the less we eat, the more cheerful we feel. But do not go to extremes. 1-2 times a week is enough to arrange fasting days, reducing the usual amount of food consumed or filling the diet only with fruits and vegetables. If you still want to experience any of the Intermittent Fasting schemes, make sure that it does not harm you. Contraindications to them are underweight – thin people cannot starve; children and old age; pregnancy and lactation; insulin-dependent diabetes mellitus; thyroid diseases, for example, thyrotoxicosis; heart rhythm disorders; myocardial infarction; heart failure; liver and kidney disease; cholelithiasis; hypotension, etc. To determine how safe starvation can be, you must consult with your doctor and pass the examinations prescribed by him. Side effects, such as constipation, headaches, dizziness, heartburn, etc., can also occur during fasting. When they appear, it is advisable to stop experimenting with oneself and smoothly go out of fasting, not snapping at food, but starting to eat gradually.

Time to starve

Many people who love to eat well, the phrase "time to starve" is not for you. You will immediately imagine a long, painful and dreary process, requiring the delivery of many tests, preliminary cleaning procedures, constant monitoring by doctors. Everything is wildly serious, scary and almost unbearable. I hasten to rejoice that in the case of Keto Diet this is absolutely not the case!

You should forget about the food, not even for a day, but only for 13–18 hours, and a significant part of this time is in sleep. This fasting can be arranged every day. If you adapt such a regime normally, then you will not have the desire to stop such a diet.

Fasting does not require special preparation, but only if you eat properly. If you are over 18 years old, you are not a pregnant woman and you are not breastfeeding, then this diet is for you. This does not require abandoning the usual physical exertion. If you, of course, are not going to run a marathon.

Of course, this also does not mean that you can have a good meal at night, go to bed and sit at the table again after 13 hours. Some conditions, though. To achieve the desired success, you should follow some rules.

   1 Dinner at least three hours before bedtime. The most ideal option, dinner 4-6 hours before bedtime, although supporters of this diet claim that 3 hours is also effective. Why is it important to observe these three hours without food?

First, almost all the calories that we consume at night are not used for their intended purpose, because during sleep, the need for energy is minimal.

Secondly, sleep is the time to detoxify and restore the body, and the need to digest food makes these processes difficult.

Thirdly, at night, we get energy from ketones, as glycogen stores begin to deplete; replenishing these reserves before bedtime does not allow the body to switch to fat burning.

2 Honest 13–18 hours of refusal to eat. More precisely, on the contrary: 18–13 hours. In this case, one should not go from the least to the most, but vice versa. Why is the recommended fasting duration exactly like that? It's simple: this is the time in which the same reserves of glycogen are consumed. What happens in 18 hours? If your body uses carbohydrates as the main fuel. Or 13 hours in the case of a low-carb diet. As for me, I started from a 13-hour fast (18 hours is still too long for me), but only after I realized that I was confidently sitting on Keto Diet.

Flexible diet schedule

From time to time, take the day off. For example, you go to an important family meal or, say, a restaurant. I consider that it is impolite to refuse to eat in such situations, and in the second case it's also stupid (why should we even go at all?). You just need to stick to the list of allowed products with Keto Diet, so as not to bring all achievements to naught.

Vary the time of the beginning and end of the fasting period. The main thing is to observe the total number of hours. That is, if I have dinner at 19.00, then I can have breakfast at 8 am. After eating at 21.00 (on the condition that I would go to bed not before midnight), I would start eating at 10 am. One of my friends, due to her occupation, cannot refuse dinner, but she never eats breakfast and begins the day with lunch. However, in the morning we often meet her for a cup of coffee. After all, with Keto Diet, breakfast means eating solid food (we recall that these are usually egg dishes, and if this is not enough, then another half avocado), so coffee, even with cream, is not considered.

The feeling of hunger can always be muffled by a cup of coffee.

No need to count calories. As in the case of some other schemes, which imply a gradual or alternate reduction. Calorie counting can be ineffective, as this is an easy mistake to make.

Drink more. As you have probably already realized, Keto Diet-starvation does not require the abandonment of all fluids at once! In this case, starving in the water does not at all mean drinking only water.

Allowed

Tea - in unlimited quantities. You can squeeze a slice of lemon into a cup.

Coffee - up to six cups per day. And in tea and coffee, you can add cream, coconut milk or butter, butter, ghee (all organic, pasteurized, not more than one tablespoon), ground cinnamon.

Chicken, fish or beef broth, in the preparation of which you can use Himalayan salt, spices, any vegetables growing above the ground, especially leafy ones, onions or shallots, carrots. Then the vegetables will have to be removed. But whole flax seeds, at the rate of one tablespoon per cup of broth, you can, on the contrary, add. Both can be drunk in unlimited quantities after you get used to fasting. It will be required less and less.

Water. So much water. In which you can sometimes throw a slice of lemon or lime (fruit do not eat) or a pinch of Himalayan salt

Contraindications to fasting and keto diet

In case of dysfunction of the adrenal glands, chronic renal diseases, chronic stress (adrenal fatigue), cortisol dysregulation, it is necessary to eliminate these disorders before embarking on fasting. This fasting is also not recommended for people with malnutrition, those who have low body weight (index less than 18.5) and who are suffering from eating disorders, including anorexia nervosa.

In addition, during fasting, avoid symptoms of hypoglycemia, or low sugar, such as dizziness, trembling, anxiety, fainting, sweating, blurred vision, slurred speech, arrhythmia, tingling of the tips of the fingers.

Chapter : 6
The Right Mindset

It really doesn't matter whether you are a newbie to intermittent fasting or you've been at it for a while. Each day you struggle to the finishing post, to the small window of time when you can eat but it seems that everywhere you look, people are eating delicious meals and sipping on full-fat flavored coffees. You find yourself resenting them while you sit and sip on a black coffee or a bottle of water, counting down the minutes and hours until you can eat again. Is that you? Most people who do on intermittent fast go through exactly the same thing but there is one way to get over it and that is to change your mindset and build up good healthy habits.

It's very easy to fall into the trap of thinking in a certain way. Many people who have tried dieting find themselves in a diet mindset – you are either on one or you aren't. You are either being good or you are cheating on your diet. And, it follows, that you are either losing weight or gaining it.

The same goes for intermittent fasting. You will, without a doubt, go at it with the same mindset – you'll reach your goal and then you'll work out how to maintain it. The biggest problem is that too many people see intermittent fasting as a temporary fix to the temporary problem of weight gain. The actual problem is in mindset. You must learn to see intermittent fasting as a permanent way of life and the only way to fix your mindset is to change it permanently. You need to shed the diet mindset and then you will start to see the results you want. You are no longer on a diet, there is no longer a point at which you stop. This is for life and the sooner you realize that, the easier it will become.

Now, this is the most important part of all. You will find yourself in another mindset – the 'can't' mindset. I can't eat until 6 pm. I can't eat when everyone else is easting. I can't add cream and sugar to my coffee. Instead of focusing on enjoying your lifestyle, you will be focusing on what you see as deprivation. Instead of thinking about what you can do, you constantly think about what you can't do.

This is the mindset you need to shake off quickly because, until you do, you can't even enjoy intermittent fasting and, believe me, it is an enjoyable lifestyle.

Instead of telling yourself that you deserve to eat when everyone else is, you need to tell yourself that you deserve your health and you deserve to lose weight more. Make that change and you'll find yourself cooking for your family without even thinking about whether you can eat or not.

How do you conquer the 'can't' mindset? How easy is it? Some people will find it easier than others but the one thing you should do is read and re-read the benefits of doing intermittent fasting. Weight loss may be your goal, but intermittent fasting is about so much more. It's about cleansing your body and slowing the aging process. It's about improving your health and having more energy. It's about rediscovering yourself, the person that you are meant to be.

You need to understand that it has nothing to do with not being able to eat when you want; it's all about choosing not to. It's about choosing to understand that your body doesn't need that much food. It's about understanding that your body will benefit from you eating the right foods but giving your body a chance to recuperate and recover every day. It's about watching the fat melt away with just one simple change to your life. Where's the hardship in that? Where's the deprivation when you find yourself fitting into clothes you never thought you'd ever be able to wear again?

The only thing you are "depriving" yourself of is bad health.

So, are you ready to make a huge change in your life? Change your mindset and you'll be happier and healthier than you ever knew. And this all leads to something else – a change in your eating habits.

Because you can only eat during a certain window of time, you'll want to make the most of it. By feeding your body healthy nutritious and delicious foods, you won't want to go back to eating junk. Sure, you can 'treat' yourself occasionally, but I promise you this – after a while on intermittent fasting, once your body gets used to eating a healthier diet, you won't want those treats.

One more thing you need to understand – this won't happen overnight. You have to work at changing both your mindset and your habits so be patient and give yourself time.

Chapter : 7
Building Muscle with Intermittent Fasting

If you combine Intermittent Fasting and high-intensity loads, you get an effective way to "dry out" the body and gain lean muscle mass. At first, of course, training on an "empty stomach" will be difficult, but our body has high adaptability. Very soon the body will get used to extracting energy not only from the usual sources (carbohydrates) but also to use this for the process of burning fat, which is required.

In conditions when the cells lack energy and at the same time the anaerobic load on the body is carried out, you get the opportunity to "start" slow muscle fibers into work (they are responsible for static long-lasting loads), thus not only getting rid of fat deposits but also increasing endurance.

If the strength training occurred during the meal, the load is best in the morning on an empty stomach; the first meal is carried out 1.5 hours after the session.

In the case when the occupation falls during the period of refusal from food, considering the low level of sugar in the blood, it is necessary to increase the rest periods between approaches and reduce weight by 15-20%. Also, be sure to use insurance.

Intermittent Fasting and Drying the body

You already imagine what periodic fasting is. The term "Drying the body" is probably familiar to you too.

The most popular ways to lose weight in sports – a low carbohydrate diet, a keto diet and the rest – are based on the principles of fractional nutrition, which periodical starvation contradicts.

The 16/8 scheme is considered optimal for Drying the body. The results of losing weight will be better if you combine the regime with proper nutrition. The only question that remains is how best to combine fasting with workouts.

Taking this table as a basis, a person with any type of employment will find the best option for himself. In addition, we recommend an excellent technique for drying the body for girls.

Diet and exercise

Morning workout

If you have a workout in the morning, then the approximate mode of your day will look like this: 6-7 a.m. training, then

12:00 p.m. first meal, then 4:30 pm. a second meal and third and last meal 8:00 p.m.

Training afternoon

If you prefer to train during the day, then you will have this mode of the day: 12:00 p.m. the first meal, then at 3:00 p.m. training, then at 4:30 pm the second meal and the last meal at 8:00 p.m.

Training in the evening

If you like evening sports, then you will have the following day regimen: at 12:00 p.m. 1st meal, 4:30 pm 2nd meal 6:00 p.m. training and then at 8:00 p.m. 3rd meal

Balanced nutrition

If you decide to lose weight while actively playing sports, you should remember that the chemical balance of Intermittent Fasting must be complete. Your diet should include the right amount of protein, fat, and carbohydrates, vitamins and minerals.

At the same time, there are some features of this kind of diet, if you want to not only lose weight but also to increase muscle mass

- If you take anabolic steroids, you need to eat more. Without the required amount of carbohydrates and protein, progress in gaining muscle mass is impossible. But at the same time, it is important that the building material is evenly ingested throughout the day, and this is almost impossible on Intermittent Fasting. It is possible to combine this type of diet with anabolic steroids only if we are talking about low dosages.

- Clenbuterol is known for its ability to transfer the body from carbohydrate to fatty energy, so the drug can be called an excellent supplement for Intermittent Fasting. In addition, it has some anti-catabolic effect.

- Bromocriptine is involved in the process of accumulating and burning fat, but it must be used correctly. Best under the guidance of an experienced coach.

Chapter : 8 How to Learn to Eating Well with Intermittent Fasting

Moving forward, as we get ever closer to our goal of completely changing our outlook on the diet, we find ourselves with a bit of an appetite. But what foods are okay to eat while fasting? Although you could safely keep your normal diet and simply fast around it, we can optimize our transformation by including foods that are ideal to pair with a diet that includes regular Intermittent Fasting. With access to nearly any food we desire, it is tough not to grab the pizza slice or burger when we feel hungry. However, we're developing our confidence and control here, not simply fulfilling our immediate desires. By taking control of our instant desires, we empower ourselves to think mindfully of our next meal, and a dedicated IF regime assists us in accomplishing this life-altering goal.

First things first, let's take a moment to think about our diets. Go back one week and write out all the meals you had including snacks and contemplate it:

Were these foods I desired? Were these foods of convenience? Were there any foods that could have been easily left out? Were these foods rich in nutrients?

These questions are pretty straightforward, but let's try and be more abstract:

Where did the food come from? Was this food natural? What time of the day was I eating? Was it a set routine? Why did I choose these particular foods? Was this the same diet I've maintained for over a decade?

This contemplation should be thorough and invigorating. There will be realizations and even more questions, more intimate ones. Let the thought process flow over you. This is a beginning step to being mindful of your diet. These simple questions will help prepare you for how your diet will change once IF begins. You will consciously change your habits, but you will also subconsciously be building a relationship with your desires and changing them from the inside out. Keep your diet in mind leading up to the fast and consider some options below if they haven't been in your diet before.

Many fad diets come and go over the years, but in reality, they are just that – fads. Cutting out carbs or only eating protein isn't going to give us the well-rounded, transformative effect we're searching for here. We need to balance our diet, explore nutrient-rich ingredients, and find alternatives to the ingredients that are most detrimental to our goals.

Moving forward, let us investigate what type of diets are best suited for IF. Since it requires you only to eat during certain parts of the day or only on certain days, we need not to just stuff ourselves with whatever we get our hands on but to be mindful of how balanced our meals are. Since we aim to lose weight while simultaneously transforming the way we view meals and food, we need meals and snacks that are mostly unprocessed, high in fiber, and have lean protein. But what we eat isn't the only factor. If you think about a 'normal' day of eating, you will realize that our digestive system is working from morning until night to digest three or more meals a day. This is just asking for weight gain since our stomachs are never empty, and our body doesn't need to burn our fat reserves for energy. So, we soon realize that the time we eat is also important. The timing will be covered in subsequent chapters.

As we think about raw, nutrient-rich food, we also consider where our food comes from. Foods produced locally will be richer in nutrients and promote the local economy by supporting smaller farms. This is a practice in mindfulness as we seek to develop a better relationship with food and, through this mindful notion, contribute to a more ecologically and economically balanced world around us. Since we seek to better ourselves through transformation, our relationship with food needs to be reevaluated, and an excellent place to start is where your food is sourced. You will also learn more about the foods available to you, educating yourself on which foods are in the season, thus helping you decide what foods you will be preparing during fasting weeks. Taking a visit to your local farmer's market is more than likely the best option for sourcing local foods, not to mention the relationship you build with other people who share the same notion of community support.

Here are some foods that are rich in nutrients and are ideal for a fasting lifestyle:

Leafy Greens

Deep, dark, leafy greens are a staple in the optimized fasting diet. These foods are rich in vitamins A, C, and K as well as plenty of potassium and fiber. These greens can replace the standard lettuce in any recipe and are available all year round. Kale, among many other leafy greens, is even considered one of the most nutrient-rich foods known to humans. If you are not a fan of the flavor of leafy greens, blend them up in a smoothie with some fruits to mask the taste. Some examples of delicious leafy greens include kale, spinach, collard greens, chard, turnip greens, and cabbage.

Garlic

Garlic is found in many recipes and can be eaten raw if you don't mind the pungent flavor and aroma. High in B vitamins, vitamin C, calcium, copper, and selenium, this nutrient-rich food could potentially lower and balance blood pressure while also containing antibacterial and antifungal properties. Garlic can be a welcome ingredient in most meals, minced or whole.

Potatoes

Potatoes are versatile and fun to cook with. They pack a massive amount of potassium, copper, and iron while also containing a good amount of vitamins B and C. Another ideal factor for IF is how filling a potato can be. Try boiling potatoes for the most beneficial preparation method.

Tomatoes

With a wide variety of different types to choose from, tomatoes are versatile and yield many different flavors. Packed full of vitamins and minerals, these beautifully bright foods can be eaten raw by themselves or added to salads.

Broccoli

Notorious for being hated by many people, broccoli is full of vitamins C and K among other vitamins and minerals. Best steamed or eaten raw in salads.

Cauliflower

Cauliflower is an incredibly nutrient-rich food that deserves way more attention. Vitamin C, K, B12, and filled with fiber, this vegetable has much-needed minerals and small amounts of protein. Find creative recipes online or eat raw in salads.

Sunflower Seeds

An excellent source of vitamin E, these tiny seeds are great to snack on. Antioxidants, copper, phosphorous, and magnesium abound in these little seeds. Add to any salad or eat raw.

Almonds

Nuts and seeds are wonderful for snacking during IF. Almonds, in particular, pack a bunch of vitamin E, copper, magnesium, and fiber. One downside is the large number of calories, so be cautious while on a restricted caloric intake and snacking on almonds.

Blueberries

Among the many berries and their many benefits, blueberries stand out when it comes to being rich in nutrients. Although not as rich in vitamins as most vegetables, blueberries boast a wild number of antioxidants, which can protect the brain and repair cells. Throw some blueberries in a salad or snack on them raw.

Raspberries

Although a little tough to find in some places, if you can get your hands on some raspberries, you can fulfill your body's needs for vitamin C, fiber, and manganese. Eat raw, with yogurt, or in smoothies.

Chocolate

You're probably thinking of name brands of candy bars right now, but in all seriousness, dark chocolate is packed with antioxidants, fiber, iron, magnesium, and copper. Grabbing chocolate with 80% or higher cocoa content is the healthiest. Mix it with smoothies, nuts, or eat raw.

Beans

Beans, black beans, in particular, are filled with iron and protein. They are filling and great to replace red meats for protein content that is much leaner. Plenty of minerals and folic acid come along with the versatile bean. Cook in chili, burritos, or even salads.

Rice

Among other whole grains, rice is rich in fiber and small amounts of vitamins and minerals. Rice is one of the most consumed foods in the world and can be mixed and paired with almost anything. Sweet or savory, rice goes a long way when fasting. It is filling, inexpensive, and easy to cook. Pair with sautéed vegetables, fish, tofu, and beans.

Tofu

Fermented soybean doesn't sound appealing to everyone, but tofu is incredibly versatile and is a great source of lean, plant-based protein. As a great alternative to red meats and other animal proteins, tofu is a lynchpin in a vegetarian or vegan diet. Marinate and sauté with veggies or press and fry for sandwiches.

Salmon

Salmon stands out among fish as a nutrient-rich powerhouse. Filled with omega-3 fatty acids and plenty of protein, salmon also helps lower heart disease. Replace beef or other meats with salmon two to three times a week for a leaner, more nutrient-rich protein source.

Shellfish

Shellfish may be the most nutritious sea creatures we know of. Clams, oysters, and mussels, among others, rank high on the oceanic food list. Excellent sources of B12 and other vitamins, these foods also contain a ton of zinc, potassium, and iron. Consume sparingly perhaps on a celebratory night out or during other special occasions.

The foods mentioned above are some of the highest valued foods for IF. Work them into your diet as well as you can, and don't be afraid to get creative with preparation techniques. Keep note of the foods that you already have in your diet and the ones you want to add to your new diet.

Meal Prepping

Along with developing a balanced and fast-friendly diet, there are techniques to take the complicated process of preparing and cooking every meal. Meal prepping, or simply meal prep, is an excellent way to save time during busy weeks, especially if you are implementing your new IF regimen. This technique is pretty straightforward: prepare all your meals for a week and store them in a container until they are ready to use. As simple as this is, let's go over some steps that often get overlooked to get you started. We will keep this step-by-step list focused on IF for the sake of our goals.

Step #1: Decide what food you want to prep

Make a list of mostly raw or unprocessed foods that you wish to consume throughout the upcoming week. Are you having the same meal every day? Or are you switching it up day to day? Once you decide what you wish to prep, head to the grocery store and be sure to buy plenty for a week's worth of meals. Some people like to choose a calorie limit and choose meals that stay under a certain caloric intake per meal. Once you have the meals in mind, continue on.

Step#2: Choose a day to prep

Your refrigerator is stocked, and you're ready to prep. Find out when your fast begins and prepare the food the day before you start. This way, the food will stay fresh longer into your week-long fast.

Step#3: Obtain containers

You will need containers to keep your prepared meals in. Tupperware and the other storage ware you have available will suffice, but many buy containers that have divided sections for the different foods. The containers need to be airtight and BPA-free. Here's a short list of features your containers should have:

- BPA-free
- eusable
- Microwave safe
- Stackable

Once you have your containers, you can start preparing the food.

Step#4: Prepare food

It's the day before you start your fast, so take your chosen ingredients and prepare them as you wish. Divide the foods out in seven equal parts for each day of the week, and then put them in the containers and store in the refrigerator. Keep in mind that uncooked foods will keep fresh longer and also pick things that will not require any further cooking or preparation once it's time to eat. Of course, having to reheat sometimes is necessary.

Step#5: Begin your week

You have your meals ready to go, and you don't need to worry about what to eat for a whole seven days. It's a nice relief – just don't forget to bring your prepared meal with you if you leave the house!

Meal prepping is a great way to keep control of your calorie intake and organize a new IF routine. With such a structured technique, it's nearly impossible to slip up on your goals. The steps above are a great foundation for an IF week. Alter the steps and quantities as you need to according to your fasting guidelines.

Below we will recommend some foods that are perfect for meal prep. Let's discuss the main courses and recommend some suitable examples of ingredients for these times of the day. The reference guide below will be focused on mostly raw unprocessed foods.

Breakfast

Breakfast is thought to be the most important meal of the day. However, this idea is flawed because it takes an entire balanced day of food to create a healthful life. No one meal is any important than the other; they all work together to create health and fulfillment. For our purposes in this book, we want breakfast foods that will not bog us down, so avoiding meats, bread, and sugary foods is ideal. With these things in mind let's take a look at some nutrient-rich foods that are great for starting the day:

- Fruits: Yes, we're avoiding sweets, but the natural source of sugar in fruit is a world away from the refined sugars we find in breakfast cereals and processed milk. An apple on the go is simple and quick. Cutting some orange slices or melon the night before is a great way to have a quick bite in the morning. Fruits are fulfilling and bursting with flavor, so for an IF regimen they come in handy as a quick source of energy or a light snack for an empty stomach.

To be clear, we are talking about raw fruits – not jellies or preserves, not an Apple Danish. Having fruit chopped and ready to eat in the refrigerator is a great habit to get into. A huge bowl of fruit salad is exceptionally tantalizing after a long fasting day.

Preparation: raw, fruit salad, paired with peanut butter, smoothie

Acceptable fruits: apples, watermelon, honeydew, cantaloupe, oranges, clementine, cherries, bananas (although bananas have the most sugar content)

- Berries: There are plenty of common misconceptions and confusion about whether or not berries are fruits. They technically are, but we'll give them a special section all to themselves. The protocol for berries is the same as fruit: have them raw or mixed in a salad.

Preparation: raw, dried, salad, paired with other fruits, smoothie

Acceptable berries: blackberry, strawberry, blueberry

- Nuts and Seeds: Like fruits, nuts and seeds make for a quick raw snack that can easily be taken on the go. When choosing nuts, be sure to pick ones that are not covered with sugar or flavors. So, avoid chocolate-covered or honey-roasted versions. Sea-salted nuts and raw nuts are the best.

Preparation: raw or roasted, trail mix, paired with fruits, smoothie

Nutritious nuts: almonds, cashews, pistachios, pecans, pumpkin seeds, sunflower seeds, chia seed, hemp seed

- Whole Grains: There are many whole grains to choose from, and these grains offer a lot in the way of fiber and carious vitamins. It is wise to eat bread sparingly, but a nice whole grain slice will go a long way; perhaps even switch bread out for a lighter option like a tortilla. The versatility of rice is a lifesaver if you're on a budget.

Preparation: cooked into oatmeal, bread, rice dishes, paired with almost anything.

Nutritious whole grains: rice, corn, oats, quinoa

- Water: This is an obvious ingredient, but also just as the only thing you have in the morning, water is a great way to start the day. Just a couple of 8-oz glasses and you're good to go – no harm in skipping out on breakfast every once in a while.

- Eggs: With eggs in the morning, we're getting to some heavier, less ideal breakfast foods. For a leaner egg, avoid eating the yolk. But if you must have eggs and need something a little bit heavier, eggs offer a high-protein inexpensive kick-start to the day.

Preparation: soft boiled, egg white omelet with veggies

- Honorable Mention – Black Coffee: Although it's a surprise, coffee is actually very healthy for you, not to mention an awesome way to start the day with its complex flavors and caffeine content. Of course, for our purposes, we will not be adding sugar, syrups, or milk to our coffee. It is highly recommended to develop a palette for black coffee and buy yourself a coffee as organic and locally roasted as possible.

Breakfast is simple. It is not necessary to eat steak, eggs, and potatoes for breakfast to 'start your day right'. Give the body some time to ease into the day by staying light and rich in nutrients for your breakfast choices.

Lunch

Midday meals are important to those who work long days and need a much-needed break. This leads to many of us settling for fast foods and sandwiches that have little nutritional value. For those who are fasting much of the time, the first solid food intake of the day is during lunchtime, so the choices we make for this meal will influence greatly how our day turns out. Meal prepping and smoothies can save you from settling for less healthy and processed foods.

- Fruits and Berries: These two food groups are going to show up a lot, so let's get used to it. These sweet foods are great for those with a nagging sweet tooth, not to mention a great source of quick energy.

Preparation: raw, dried, salad, paired with other fruits, smoothie

Acceptable berries: blackberry, strawberry, blueberry

- Vegetables: With such a wide variety to choose from, there is a veggie for everyone. Rich in fiber and various vitamins, vegetables are an IF's best friend. We can chat all day about the variety of ways vegetables can be prepared and consumed, but for a midday meal, salad is King.

Preparation: steamed or sautéed, eaten raw or with salad

Nutritious vegetables: tomatoes, broccoli, Brussel sprouts, potatoes, kale, carrots, spinach, cauliflower

- Nuts and Seeds: Like fruits, nuts and seeds make for a quick raw snack that can easily be taken on the go. When choosing nuts, be sure to pick ones that are not covered with sugar or flavors. So, avoid chocolate-covered or honey-roasted versions. Sea-salted nuts and raw nuts are the best.

Preparation: raw or roasted, trail mix, paired with fruits, smoothie

Nutritious nuts: almonds, cashews, pistachios, pecans, pumpkin seeds, sunflower Seeds, chia seed, hemp seed

- Whole Grains: There are many different whole grains to choose from, and these grains offer a lot in the way of fiber and carious vitamins. It is wise to eat breads sparingly, but a nice whole grain slice will go a long way perhaps even switch bread out for a lighter option like a tortilla. The versatility of rice is a lifesaver if you're on a budget.

Preparation: cooked into oatmeal, bread, rice dishes, paired with almost anything.

Nutritious whole grains: rice, corn, oats, quinoa

- Chicken: Very lean and readily available, chicken is carbohydrate free and has very little fat and calorie content. It is an easy transition to cut out red meats and replace them with chicken. It's easy to prepare and versatile.

Preparation: boiled, sautéed, not breaded, tossed in a salad

Nutritious chicken: Not breaded, lightly seasoned, free range

Dinner

The last full meal of the day, dinner/supper is typically reserved for heavy meals and entertaining guests. The evening meal sets the tone of the evening and often is the meal that is most well thought out throughout the day. Steaks, burgers, and other heavy entrées rule this meal in the Western world, but we want to find leaner and more nutritious options for our purposes.

- Fish: Eating fish in place of heavier, less lean meats is a great way to alter your evening diet for the fasting lifestyle. In place of steaks, burgers, and pork, substitute the more nutrient-rich and lighter variety of fish or seafood.

Nutritious fish: salmon, albacore, sardines, trout, oysters

Preparation: Cooked thoroughly, sautéed or steam

- Chicken: Very lean, and readily available, chicken is carbohydrate free and has very little fat and calorie content. It is an easy transition to cut out red meats and replace them with chicken. It's easy to prepare and versatile.

Preparation: boiled, sautéed, not breaded

Nutritious chicken: not breaded, lightly seasoned, free range

- Tofu: The go-to replacement for meat-based protein, tofu is a soybean product that is full of great protein. It is a staple in Eastern cultures, and the Western world is slowly getting on board. Tofu is almost flavorless by itself, but when marinated or combined with veggies in a rice dish, it's just as valuable as any meat.

- Vegetables: With such a wide variety to choose from, there is a veggie for everyone. Rich in fiber and various vitamins, vegetables are an IF's best friend. We can chat all day about the variety of ways vegetables can be prepared and consumed, but for an evening meal, a salad appetizer or a sautéed side dish are winners.

Preparation: steamed or sautéed

Nutritious vegetables: tomatoes, broccoli, Brussel sprouts, potatoes, kale, carrots, spinach, cauliflower

- Whole Grains: There are many different whole grains to choose from, and these grains offer a lot in the way of fiber and carious vitamins. It is wise to eat breads sparingly, but a nice whole grain slice will go a long way, perhaps even switch bread out for a lighter option like a tortilla. The versatility of rice is a lifesaver if you're on a budget.

Preparation: cooked into oatmeal, bread, rice dishes, paired with almost anything

Nutritious whole grains: rice, corn, oats, quinoa

This basic guide to what foods are best at which part of the day is great for developing your own diet plan.

Snacks

Light snacks throughout the day help to appease your appetite and offer a much-needed break from monotonous days. Keeping snack foods handy is also a practice and also for safety – just in case your fasting days get the best of you, and you find yourself losing all your energy. Although it's popular to keep processed snacks nearby, chips, candies, and sodas are not ideal or our goals at hand.

Preparation: raw, trail mix, organic prepackaged

Nutritious snacks: nuts, seeds, fruits, veggies, granola, dark chocolate

Notable Diets

With weight loss in mind, we should explore some popular diets that pair quite well with IF. There are a few diets that have hit the mainstream and come equipped with the guidelines and structure needed to optimize weight loss when paired with IF. While diets have served as the stand-in for what it takes to be healthy in recent decades, studies have shown that simply altering what foods you eat will not lead to a healthful and balanced life. Many subtle changes need to be implemented to achieve these goals. Yes, the food you eat is very important, but it's not the end-all-be-all of healthful practices. Going on a diet for a month doesn't change your life. If you want a healthy life and wish to maintain that health, you will need to balance all aspects of health – not just the food you eat. Below we will explore some diets and how they are perfect for IF.

Mediterranean Diet

This diet is inspired by the foods and nutritional outlook of people living near the Mediterranean Sea. Fruits, legumes, vegetables, and other plant-based foods rule this diet, along with an abundant amount of extra-virgin olive oil and fresh fish.

As it is well known, the culture and societies surrounding the Mediterranean are joyous about their meals, not to mention red wines. The celebratory nature of their lifestyles is no doubt key in their health and happiness. This mindful attitude is exactly what we aim for when it comes to our own relationships with food. The positive mindset, vegetables, fresh lean protein, and plenty of healthy fats make this diet, as well as the cultures that influence it, ideal for IF.

Paleo Diet

The Paleo diet, or caveman diet, is one of the more popular diets that has seen its fifteen minutes of fame but has continued onward after its initial boom in the mainstream media. The diet is loosely based on what we think our ancient ancestors consumed before agriculture and farming was developed. As far as studies go, it is thought that our ancestors were extremely active and ate a diet of organic and wild meats, nuts, greens, and even insects.

Many assume that the prehistoric man thrived mainly on meat, but this is a common misconception. Hunting alone would not yield enough food for a large tribe, so it's commonly thought that less than half of the diet would consist of meat. The rest of the diet would be filled with foraged foods like plants, berries, seeds, and nuts. Considering different regions around the world and the vague nature of studying the past, there is a lot of difference in opinion when it comes to the Paleo diet. It is safe to say that not all hunts would be successful, so there would be prolonged instances of sustaining on nothing but plant-based foods. This pattern of eating, in essence, is IF. So, the Paleo diet has a history with IF, but how can we apply this to the modern world?

There is no one strict structure for the Paleo diet. And given the variety of diets in the ancient world, on a scale from low-carb, high animal content to high-carb plant-based, many different styles can be considered 'paleo'. So, here is a general outline for what foods to eat with a basic Paleo diet:

- Meat (fish, lamb, beef, chicken, seafood)
- Eggs (free range, cage free)

- Vegetables (potatoes, broccoli, carrots, tomatoes)
- Nuts and Seeds (almonds, walnuts, sunflower seeds, pumpkin seeds)
- Fruits (apples, pears, oranges, avocados)
- Healthy Oils (extra virgin olive oil, coconut oil)
- Herbs (sea salt, rosemary, turmeric, garlic)

This list is a great stepping stone to more specific guidelines, and keep in mind this food should be as organic as possible, and the fruits, nuts, and herbs being wild foraged, of course. For a stricter regimen, here is a list of foods to avoid:

- Legumes (beans, lentils, peanuts)
- Grains (bread, pasta, wheat, rye, barley)
- Dairy (some diets allow butter and cheese)
- Some oils (soybean, corn, sunflower, grapeseed)
- Artificial sweeteners (sucralose, aspartame)
- Very processed foods (frozen, prepackaged, additives)

Ketogenic Diets

As we discussed briefly, ketosis is when your body has used up all its quick energy and creates ketones to help burn stored fat. Typically, these diets are all about high-fat, low-carbohydrate meals, like plenty of eggs, avocados, and fatty meats, while avoiding bread and whole grains which are the prime source of carbs in the contemporary diet.

By cutting back our carbohydrate consumption to 60 grams or less per day for four to five days, our body will begin to produce ketones, which allow the body to use stored fat. The body cannot directly use the fat on its own. This diet, paired with an IF routine, can be very effective for our weight loss purposes. However, we need to take into account the dangers that ketosis can be present for certain people. Avoid inducing ketosis if you have diabetes, are taking high blood pressure medication, or breastfeeding.

Vegetarian Diets

Vegetarian diets are popular all around the world and in many countries and cultures. Even within the scope of the Paleo diet, vegetarianism is acceptable at times. The diet is not only a healthy alternative to contemporary Western diets but is also more ecologically friendly compared to a diet where all the protein comes from animal-based sources. Many vegetarians choose this diet for the health benefits and their overall wellbeing, but many people find themselves practicing this diet for their love of animals and the earth.

As you are more than likely aware, the vegetarian's diet has a strict no-meat rule. This means no beef, pork, fish, chicken, or any other meat. Many vegetarians still consume eggs, eat butter, and use milk, but strictly no meat itself is consumed. Much of the scientific motivation behind the vegetarian diet is that plant-based proteins are better for you and easier to digest than red meats. Although this diet is just as balanced as any other, when approaching a vegetarian diet, it is important that you eat plenty of protein to make up for the immense amount of protein lost when cutting out meats. Another issue is iron and sodium intake that is found abundantly in meat. These building blocks of life need extra attention with a vegetarian diet. Regardless of motivation, the vegetarian diet is great for IF, with all the nutrient-rich ingredients found in the world of animal-free sustenance.

Vegan Diet

Another animal-free diet, the vegan diet is similar to the vegetarian diet, but instead of simply cutting out meat itself, this diet requires that you cut out all animal products. Eggs, milk, butter, and anything with the slightest bit of animal-related ingredients are off limits. This an extreme version of vegetarianism and even crosses over into other territories besides the individual's diet. Many vegans take pride in their decision to avoid all animal products every moment of their lives – no fur clothing, no products tested on animals, absolutely nothing that uses animals. This diet comes with a philosophy, and here in this book, our goals are elsewhere. There is plenty of information online about veganism.

The Whole30 Diet

This diet has seen a surge in popularity in recent years with the 'gluten-free' trend that has been going around. The diet itself calls for us to eliminate foods that are common culprits when it comes to allergies and intolerances. So, it means cutting out gluten-rich grains and legumes like beans and peanuts. The diet involves a 30-day 'clean eating' cycle where you cut these potentially unhealthy foods out of your diet for 30 days, then see how you feel. You can gradually reintroduce these foods and again take note of your body's reactions. This diet can almost allow us to see if we are intolerant to certain foods, thus allowing us to cut out troublesome ingredients. This is also a great diet for developing mindfulness and awareness about our bodies. It will pair well with an IF week at the end of the 30-day cycle.

Raw Food Diet

The raw food diet is very similar to the vegan diet, and many vegans adhere to its basic principle of eating foods in their natural form. It includes raw fruits, vegetables, nuts, and seeds. Uncooked and not dehydrated or seasoned, the nutritional value of these foods in this diet cannot be debated. This diet is a pretty simple one, but it is more than likely a world away from your current diet. Some may find it difficult not to cook, and without cooking your meal choices are limited. This diet will be one of the more difficult to uphold, not to mention one of the more difficult diets to practice and also ensure that you get all the needed nutrients. However, if you feel like the raw food diet suits you, try it out and pay very close attention to what your body says in return.

With the incredible variety of diets available online, there's no shortage of plans, routines, and fads. It is best to avoid choosing a diet based on popularity and choose diets that you will actually enjoy. There's no reason to take all the joy out of eating and the art of cooking in exchange for a routine that may not even be very effective. With this in mind, we can safely say that if you find that a diet needs a little customization to suit your needs, then go ahead and alter it. This is your practice; this is your life. Take control and empower yourself regardless of what people say. Enjoyment of food and your lifestyle choices are just as important as the choices themselves. If we are not taking pleasure out of our choices, then we need to rearrange and alter our current routine.

Once we have established our preferred dietary choices or altered our diet to one with foods that are more suitable for IF, we can begin making preparations to start our fasting week.

Chapter : 8
How to set a Healthy Lifestyle with Intermittent Fasting

In our world today, the standard of beauty and what constitutes the ideal physique has promoted and even praised unrealistic expectations for men and women alike. Everywhere you look there are cover models on magazines with chiseled abs, models fitting perfectly in size zero dresses, actors in every movie with physiques the average person could probably never obtain. Being exposed to this sort of standard from every angle day after day, can most definitely wear on our self-image and confidence.

Like I said, this goes for both men and women, but I think we can all agree that women bear the brunt of this aspect of life. The media does its very best to make you believe that you cannot be considered pretty, or in shape, unless you mimic these unrealistic expectations presented to you in the magazines and television. Sadly, this not only leads to lowered self-esteem in large numbers of women, but sometimes it can escalate into health disorders.

To try and cope with these expectations, some individuals develop a severe eating disorder known as bulimia. This is a disorder where someone consumes usually a large amount of food, feels guilty, and then becomes so worried that it will be detrimental to their physique that they actually induce vomiting, or take a large amount of laxatives, in a desperate attempt to reverse the situation. These methods are usually referred to as "purging." This disorder can wreak absolute havoc on the body. People with bulimia commonly have severe stomach distortion from overeating, electrolyte imbalance from severe dehydration, ulcers covering the lining of their esophagus from the constant stomach acid coming up from vomiting, and tooth decay also due to stomach acid. Although men and women both suffer from this disorder, women are much more prone to it. The United States Department of Health and Human Services reports that as many as 2% of women suffer from this eating disorder.

Another severe eating disorder many people suffer from is anorexia. This results in a person limiting their food intake to dangerously low levels for fear of gaining weight, exercising far too much in an attempt to burn calories. They often have a severely distorted body image in which they feel that their obese, when in reality they are far too thin. Once again, even though this disorder affects both men and women, it is predominately a female condition, with an estimated 1 in 20 women in the United States suffering from anorexia. This disorder also has terrible health implications such as heart problems, anemia, and extremely high-risk pregnancies.

Eating disorders are a real problem, and women are overwhelmingly more prone to developing them. So, how does all of this information relate to intermittent fasting, you may wonder? Well, my point is that with the way intermittent fasting places on emphasis on specific periods of fasting, followed by strict eating windows, it can sometimes cause women to develop an unhealthy obsession with food.

If your body is still getting used to going extended periods of time without eating, there is a greater likelihood that when the feeding window begins you will be so hungry that you overdo it. If you are really wanting to see results from following this protocol and are ashamed of yourself for consuming an excessive amount of food, the guilt you feel might even lead you to becoming bulimic, purging yourself to try and undo the situation. Likewise, if after adhering to intermittent fasting for some time and not seeing the results that you hoped for, you may start to feel like what you are doing is not enough. This can cause women to become more predisposed to developing anorexia.

When this happens, it is easy to see how someone may shorten their eating window far too much, or barely eat any food at all during the allotted feeding time. Although women must be aware and cautious of these eating disorders when beginning intermittent fasting, this becomes even more important if they have any prior history of eating disorders, as the likelihood of relapsing increases substantially. To prevent any of these eating disorders from rearing their ugly head, one needs to make sure that their perspective is in the right place. The first thing you need to remember is that intermittent fasting is about becoming a healthier, happier version of you.

Remember all of the benefits you can enjoy that we discussed earlier? Well these don't mean anything if you develop an extremely unhealthy relationship with food in the process. It is important that you keep in mind why you started it in the first place; to better yourself. The second thing to keep in mind is that you are a human being (shocker, right?). We are imperfect creatures with limited self-control, we make mistakes.

I can assure you that if you choose to begin intermittent fasting, there will be times that you make mistakes. Maybe that eating window just cannot wait, and you give in to the hot and ready sign at Krispy Kreme on your way home. Sometimes you may consume a few too many calories when those precious feeding hours begin. In nutrition, fitness, and even life in general, it is never the small, infrequent things that yield long term results. What you need to remember is that the things you do HABITUALLY are what will make or break you.

If you eat a terrible diet routinely and randomly decide to eat healthy for only one day, do you think you are going to immediately lose 10 pounds? Is going to the gym twice a year going to get you in fantastic shape and allow you to reach your fitness goals? Having said that, slipping up on your diet from time to time or missing a workout every once in a while, is not going to ruin your weight-loss and exercise goals. Anything worth achieving, especially when it comes to your body, is not going to happen overnight.

However, if you consistently follow the intermittent fasting protocol, or any other diet for that matter, then even with the minor setbacks that happen you are still on the path to your goals! When it comes to intermittent fasting, you need to understand that this is merely a tool at your disposal that you are choosing to use to become a healthier person. You must never let something like this control you, after all, you are the one in control choosing to live this lifestyle, and you have the power to stop or change the rules at any time.

In your journey with intermittent fasting, it is of the utmost importance that you never lose sight of the big picture. Remember that food is not the most important thing in your life, and preoccupation with eating should never get in the way of the things that matter most to you. Although cruel, societal definitions and images portrayed by the media are giving us a horrible definition of what it means to be healthy.

Most of the muscular men shown in movies and magazine covers are abusing harmful substances such as anabolic steroids, and a large number of women modeling the latest fashions are secretly suffering from the eating disorders that we discussed.

If you let it, comparing yourself to these people will do nothing but rob you of your joy and discourage you from trying to be your best. The only measuring stick that you should stand next to in your journey should be your former self. It is amazing how much fitness and nutrition mirror all of life itself. In everything you do, you should wake up every morning trying to improve yourself from the you that fell asleep last night. Never let anyone tell you that you are not good enough and that you're not capable of reaching your health and wellness goals. You are more than capable of achieving them with the right amount of knowledge and commitment.

Chapter : 9
How to Heal your Body with Intermittent Fasting

When it comes to female hormones, reproductive health takes internal and unspoken precedence over the weight concerns of the conscious individual. This primacy of reproductive health stands out more so with females than it does with males, as we discovered in the last chapter through the 2013 rat studies and more. However, there have to be bigger biological reasons behind that increased sensitivity.

The cause seems to be kisspeptin, which is a molecule similar to a protein that helps neurons communicate with each other about hunger and energy and more. This molecule exists in both males and females, but females have far more kisspeptin than males do, making them even more sensitive to energetic changes in their internal balances.

Therefore, when females' bodies release hormones like leptin, ghrelin, and insulin (that make them feel hungry or full), their brains and internal systems are already that much more inclined to "hear" those feelings and respond to reestablish balance. Women are therefore more likely to struggle with weight loss and general health problems related to increased sensitivity. Despite your body's natural processes, however,

120

you can *absolutely* learn how to make intermittent fasting work for you and still maintain your ideal weight, health, and productivity.

Using IF to Help with Periods, Fertility, and Metabolism

If you struggle monthly through painful periods; if you know you don't want to have children and you're not concerned about future fertility; or if you want to kick-start your metabolism to help yourself lose weight, all you have to do is start intermittently fasting without any concern whatsoever. If you're looking for hard and fast changes for your harsh menses, your fertility, or your weight issues, work your way up to fasting a few days a week, and you're sure to see the side-effects you seek played out within a month or two.

If you're interested in getting help with painful periods without substantial effects on your future fertility, simply make sure to get enough fat in your diet and supplemental estrogen (which you can find over the counter in a variety of forms). By making sure to consume enough healthy fat and by not restricting your caloric intake too much, you can use intermittent fasting to ease difficult menses without it having too much effect on your metabolism at the moment, and with it having hardly any effect on your fertility later on.

If you want the metabolism boost without effect on your periods or fertility, here's what you can do. Make sure you're eating enough healthy fats, but restrict caloric intake slightly, not too much though, mind you! You don't want to hurt those hunger hormones or inhibit your ability to ovulate and have a healthy period!

For these reasons, you should make sure *not* to intentionally or fastidiously "diet" while you're intermittently fasting but seeing as how you *do* want to lose weight and kick-start that metabolism, you can do *something* to help your body remember not to hang onto too much excess! That *"something"* that works so well is two-part: (1) once you define your method, keep to its timing strictly and; (2) when you have your meals, don't overindulge, binge, or gorge yourself; allow your caloric intake to be limited, but only slightly, as you work with IF.

Chapter : 10
Tips for Intermittent Fasting

You must not avoid eating vegetables. Make sure that 75% of your minimum carbohydrate intake comes from vegetables. This means that you must eat at least two cups of cooked vegetables and up to 6 cups of leafy vegetables per day.

Drink Plenty of Water

You must drink at least 8 cups of water a day. This can increase with increasing physical activity. As long as your urine is pale or clear, it means you are drinking enough water. Two cups can be in the form of coffee or tea, broth or drinks without sugar. Don't make the terrible mistake of drinking less water. If you do not drink enough water, your body will start retaining water, and it will lead to weight gain. Drink plenty of water to prevent dehydration. During intermittent fasting, you must not eat food while fasting. Water will help prevent any hunger pangs. Not only that, it makes your skin younger and fresher. You can add a few pieces of lemon and a sprig of mint to spruce up your regular water.

Don't be Scared of Fats

Certain dietary fats are necessary for the body to burn fat, and these natural fats are good if you remember your carbohydrate intake. You must always accompany the undershot carbohydrates with fats or proteins.

Consumption of Hidden Carbs

Carefully read the labels on the packaged foods you consume. Just because the package says it's low in calories, please don't think that this means low carbohydrate content. Make sure you use full-fat mayonnaise, salad dressings, and other similar products. Low-fat varieties tend to mix extra sugar to replace the taste of butter.

Record your Progress

You must never forget to record your progress. Keep a journal for all your weekly records of your weight and measurements. You can also turn on the food log to track the number of carbohydrates consumed. As you follow your progress, you can make the necessary changes to your diet to make it a good fit with your metabolism. Several calorie-counting apps let you track the number of calories consumed.

Plan your Meals

On the days of fasting, you must plan your meals in advance. It will be quite annoying if you had to feverishly search your office or home to find something to eat, won't it? It is likely that everything you find is full of sugar or contains processed carbohydrates. Such food will make you hungry within no time, and it is not good for you as well. So, if you know in advance what you can eat and how many calories the food makes, it's easier to follow a diet. It also keeps you from giving in to temptation.

Lots of Protein

Protein helps you to feel full for a long time. Eggs are a good option. Adding an egg to your meal can make a big difference. It not only provides you with extra energy but it also makes you feel fuller. You can add any form of lean meat to your meals and even opt for protein shakes. As long as your calorie intake is in the range of 500 to 600, everything is fine. This does not mean that you must consume only protein and omit vegetables or vice versa. This has a negative effect on your weight loss, and you also feel strong cravings for carbohydrates.

Include Fiber in Meals

One of the most attractive things about this diet is the flexibility it offers. There are no hard and fast rules about the food you can consume, but it doesn't mean that you consume all sorts of unhealthy foods. So, what can one eat when following intermittent fasting? Ensuring a healthy diet is necessary. The minimum calorie intake must be over 1200 calories, and all these calories go into the body's hunger mode. If you are a woman, you must value fiber and dietary fats.

Fibrous food is not only useful for you but also to make you feel full longer. You can have green leafy vegetables. They take more time to digest than carbs and contain fewer calories. The combination of lean protein and a large portion of vegetables will help you survive your contribution.

Drink Tea or Black Coffee

On days of fasting, you can drink lots of green or black tea. The warm water will fill your tummy, and the caffeine helps suppress your appetite; however, keep away from any prepackaged drinks. You can also consume black coffee without adding any sugar or cream to it. Having a cup of black coffee in the morning on the days of fast will help curb hunger and make you feel energetic; however, ensure that you don't consume too much of caffeine since it has a diuretic effect on the body.

Tips to Stay Motivated

Now that you know the different forms of intermittent fasting and the tips you can follow to lose weight, the next step is to start with this diet. Have you ever tried a diet before? Are you afraid that you will lose motivation in a few weeks? If you want to reach your health and fitness goals, make sure your mojo does not hesitate. Motivation gives you the strength you need to stick to your diet and overcome potential difficulties. In this section, you will learn some simple tips that you can follow, so that your motivation never hesitates.

Set realistic goals

If you do not want your motivation to slow down after starting a diet, it is very important that you set yourself realistic goals before starting a diet. Setting goals are important in all areas of your life, and this also applies to your diet. Your goals must be not only achievable but also realistic. If you set unattainable goals, you will be doomed to fail. For instance, if your goal of losing weight is to lose 30 pounds in a month, this is not practical. This is not only inappropriate, but it isn't healthy. If you set yourself such a goal, you are simply ready to fail. Instead, it makes sense to set a practical goal, such as losing 30 pounds in about 8-10 weeks. If you want to lose weight and make sure that weight loss is stable over the long term.

Slow down

If you want a diet to be effective, it will mainly depend on your lifestyle. The diet will generate positive results, but it takes some time. Such changes take some time, and you will not notice success overnight. If you want to lose weight, maintain the weight loss, and stick to the diet in the long run, it's a good idea to lose weight slowly. Of course, you can starve yourself and lose a few pounds within a week, but this weight loss is not sustainable. A sudden drop in the balance is undesirable compared to a permanent weight reduction. Intermittent fasting is a great diet, and it is stable. Slow and steady wins the race, and it cannot be more apt for intermittent fasting.

Expect some Setbacks

Failures are a part of life, and some of them are to be expected, even if you follow a new diet. Temptation can strike anyone. There will be times when you want to and can give in to your temptations. There is no damage to it, and some slipups are common. The real problem occurs when you use such instances as an excuse for overeating. If you think, "Well, I still broke my diet, so it's okay if I ate that bag of chips," then you'll be in a world of trouble. If you think that way, you will have unnecessary problems. You need to remember that you are only a human being and that failure is part of life. Learn to deal with a mistake and always treat it as an isolated case. If you ignore your diet on one day, treat it as an isolated incident and return to your diet from the next day. It's okay to experience setbacks, but the real problem starts when you think of them as a failure. The attitude you follow in dealing with such failures is very important.

Don't be a perfectionist

All right, let's say you binged on a pint of ice cream. What will you do? Thinking like a perfectionist will do you more harm than good. If you feel that consuming 2000 calories is nothing but indulgence, you are safe; however, if you think that this is a failure and the reason for stopping the diet, a 1500-calorie snack can quickly become a 4000-calorie snack. Do not try to be a perfectionist, especially if you are dieting.

Chapter : 11
Recipes for Weight Loss with Intermittent Fasting

Breakfast

1. Chicken Breakfast Muffins

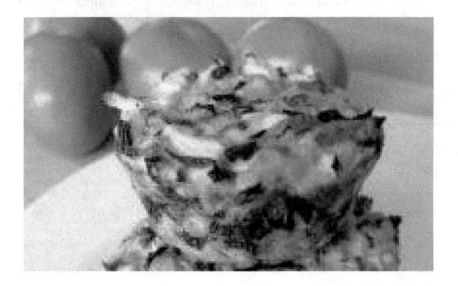

Ingredients:

- ¾ pound chicken breast, boneless
- Salt and ground black pepper, to taste
- ½ teaspoon garlic powder
- 3 tablespoons hot sauce mixed with 3 tablespoons melted coconut oil
- 6 eggs

- 2 tablespoons green onions, chopped

Directions:

Season the chicken breast with salt, pepper, and garlic powder, place it on a lined baking sheet and bake in the oven at 425°F for 25 minutes. Transfer the chicken breast to a bowl, shred with a fork, and mix with half of the hot sauce and melted coconut oil. Toss to coat, and set aside. In a bowl, mix the eggs with salt, pepper, green onions, and the rest of the hot sauce mixed with oil and whisk. Divide this mixture into a muffin tray, top each with shredded chicken, place in an oven at 350°F, and bake for 30 minutes. Serve the muffins hot.

Nutrition: Calories - 140, Fat - 8, Fiber - 1, Carbs - 2, Protein - 13

2. **Breakfast Muffins**

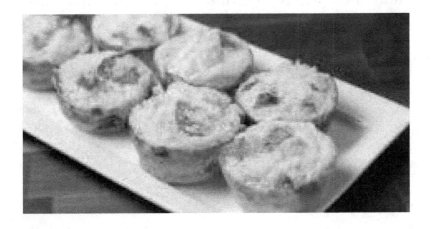

Preparation time: 10 minutes

Cooking time: 30 minutes

Servings: 4

Ingredients:

- ½ cup almond milk
- 6 eggs
- 1 tablespoon coconut oil
- Salt and ground black pepper, to taste
- ¼ cup kale, chopped
- 8 prosciutto slices
- ¼ cup fresh chives, chopped

Directions:

In a bowl, mix the eggs with salt, pepper, milk, chives, and kale. Grease a muffin tray with melted coconut oil, line with prosciutto slices, pour the eggs mixture, place in an oven, and bake at 350°F for 30 minutes. Transfer muffins to a platter, and serve.

Nutrition: Calories - 140, Fat - 3, Fiber - 1, Carbs - 3, Protein - 10

3. Breadless Breakfast Sandwich

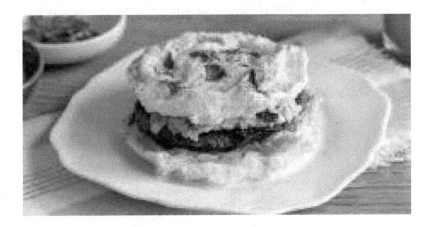

Preparation time: 10 minutes

Cooking time: 10 minutes

Servings: 1

Ingredients:

- 2 eggs
- Salt and ground black pepper, to taste
- 2 tablespoons butter
- ¼ pound pork sausage, minced
- ¼ cup water
- 1 tablespoon guacamole

Directions:

In a bowl, mix the minced sausage meat with some salt and pepper, and stir well. Shape a patty from this mixture and place it on a working surface. Heat up a pan with 1 tablespoon butter over medium heat, add the sausage patty, fry for 3 minutes on each side, and transfer to a plate. Crack an egg into 2 bowls and whisk them with some salt and pepper. Heat up a pan with the rest of the butter over medium-high heat, place 2 biscuit cutters that you've greased with some butter in the pan and add an egg to each one. Add the water to the pan, reduce heat, cover pan, and cook eggs for 3 minutes. Transfer these egg "buns" to paper towels and drain the excess grease.

Place sausage patty on one egg "bun," spread guacamole over it, and top with the other egg "bun,"

Nutrition: Calories - 200, Fat - 4, Fiber - 6, Carbs - 5, Protein - 10

4. Vegetable Breakfast Bread

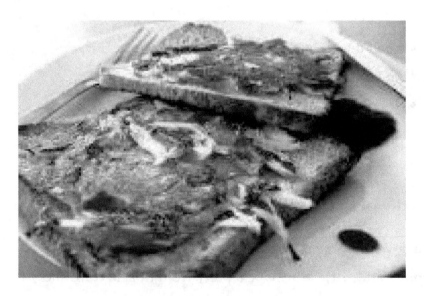

Preparation time: 10 minutes

Cooking time: 25 minutes

Servings: 7

Ingredients:

- 1 cauliflower head, separated into florets
- ½ cup fresh parsley, chopped
- 1 cup spinach, torn
- 1 onion, peeled and chopped
- 1 tablespoon coconut oil
- ½ cup pecans, ground
- 3 eggs
- 2 garlic cloves, peeled and minced
- Salt and ground black pepper, to taste

Directions:

In a food processor, mix the cauliflower florets with some salt, and pepper, and pulse well. Heat up a pan with the oil over medium heat, add the cauliflower, onion, and garlic, some salt and pepper, stir, and cook for 10 minutes. In a bowl, mix the eggs with salt, pepper, parsley, spinach, and nuts, and stir. Add the cauliflower mixture, and stir well. Spread this mixture into forms placed on a baking sheet, heat oven to 350°F, and bake for 15 minutes. Serve warm.

Nutrition: Calories - 140, Fat - 3, Fiber - 3, Carbs - 4, Protein - 8

Lunch

1 Albacore Tuna Vinaigrette Salad

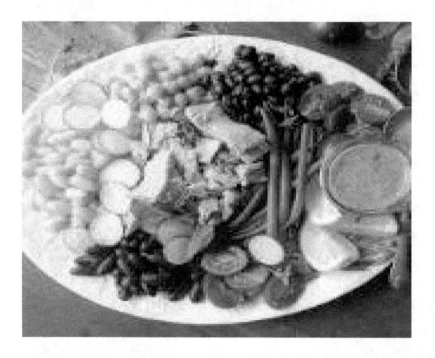

Prep time: 10 min;

Cook time: 7 min

Serving Size: 1/4;

Serves: 4;

Calories: 231

Total Fat: 20g;

Protein: 9g;

Total Carbs: 5.5g

Dietary Fiber: 5g;

Sugar: 0g;

Sodium: 265mg

Ingredients

- 1 can albacore tuna, drained
- 1 pound of fresh or frozen asparagus
- ¼ cup walnuts, chopped
- cups baby salad mix
- ½ tsp salt
- ¼ tsp pepper
- tsp finely chopped onion
- 1 tsp spicy brown mustard
- tsp wine vinegar, white or red
- ¼ cup olive oil or garlic sesame oil
- 1 Splenda packet

Directions

Mix together the spices and the tuna, set aside.

Steam the asparagus for 5-7 minutes until desired crispness.

Place the salad mixture onto 4 plates.

Divide the asparagus by 4 and place on salad greens.

Divide the seasoned tuna by 4 and scatter onto the asparagus and salad.

Sprinkle each salad with the walnuts and serve.

Prep Instructions

Place the tuna mixture in a zip-lock bag and place in the fridge. Steam the asparagus and place in a zip-lock bag in the fridge. Place the salad mix in zip-locks in the fridge. Put the walnuts in a bag in the fridge.

2   Barbecue Chicken Pizza

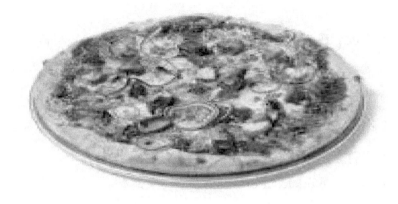

Prep time: 19 min;

Cook time: 29 min

Serving Size: 1 pizza;

Serves: 8

Calories: 285

Total Fat: 12g;

Protein: 27g

Total Carbs: 7g

Dietary Fiber: 5g;

Sugar: 0g;

Sodium: 100mg

Ingredients

- 1/2 cup G Hughes Smokehouse BBQ Sauce, sugar free
- ½ tsp salt
- cups baking mix, low-carb
- 1 cup water
- 1 chopped red onion
- 1 cup cooked chicken, diced
- ½ cup chopped bell peppers, red, green, yellow assortment
- ½ cup sliced black olives
- T olive oil
- 1 cup mozzarella cheese, hand-shredded
- ½ c parmesan cheese, hand-shredded
- 1 packet Splenda or sweetener of your choice

Directions

Set oven to 425 F.

Mix into a dough the baking powder, baking mix, Splenda, salt, water, and oil.

Place of waxed paper and lightly oil. Roll into your pizza crust.

Bake for 9 minutes.

Remove from heat source and spread the barbecue sauce onto the crust.

Layer the toppings, placing the cheeses on top.

Bake 15 more minutes until thoroughly warmed and the cheese is melted.

Slice into 8 pieces and serve.

Freezing Directions

Place individual slices in a zip-lock freezer bag. Freeze. To serve, heat in microwave one minute.

3   Bok-Choy Ginger Soup

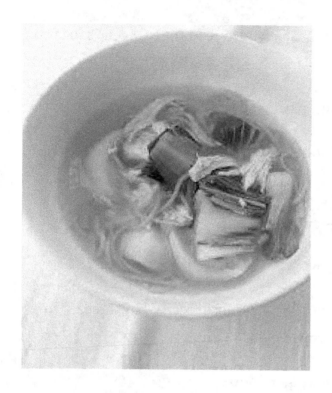

Prep time: 9 min;

Cook time: 9 min;

Serving Size: 1 cup;

Serves: 4;

Calories: 65

Total Fat: 2g;

Protein: 7g;

Total Carbs: 5g

Dietary Fiber: 2g;

Sugar: 0g;

Sodium: 100mg

Ingredients

- cups diced green onions
- cups chopped or sliced mushrooms
- tsp fresh grated ginger
- tsp minced garlic
- T tamari
- 2 cups chopped bok-choy
- 1 T cilantro, chopped
- oz. firm tofu, cut into bite sized squares
- 3 T grated carrot
- 1 can diced tomatoes and peppers
- cups chicken broth

Directions

Place everything but the green onions, tofu, and carrot into a sauce and bring to a boil.

Reduce the heat to low-med and cook this for 6 minutes.

Stir in the green onions, tofu, and carrots. Cook for 2 more minutes.

Serve sprinkled with the cilantro.

Freezing Instructions

Let soup cool thoroughly. Pour into four containers that have lids. Freeze. Microwave 2-3 minutes to serve.

4 Chicken Lettuce Wraps

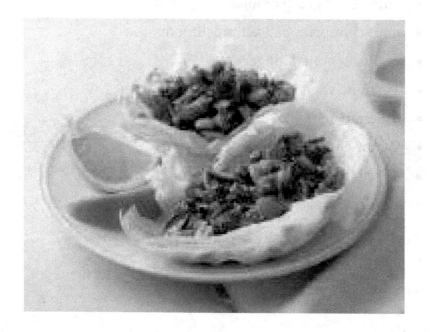

Prep time: 10min;

Cook time: 10min

Serving Size: 1;

Serves: 1;

Calories: 145

Total Fat: 1g;

Protein: 35g;

Dietary Fiber: 1g;

Total Carbs: 4g

Sugar: 0g;

Sodium: 100mg

Ingredients

- 1 chicken breast, boneless, diced into 1-inch size pieces
- 1 cup diced or sliced fresh mushrooms
- ½ cup diced water chestnuts (from a can, drained)
- 1 T olive oil
- 1 T onion, minced
- 1 T minced garlic
- 1 T teriyaki sauce
- garlic powder, only a dash
- onion powder, just a dash
- oregano, one dash
- cayenne pepper, a small dash
- salt / pepper

Directions

Mix the ingredients and cook in a skillet until the chicken is done, about 10 minutes.

Shred the chicken

Place in leaves and roll

Freezing Instructions

Place all ingredients into one freezer bag except the lettuce. Microwave one minute and serve.

5   Chicken Quesadillas

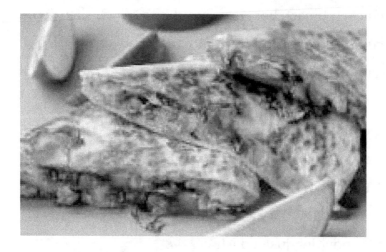

Prep time: 4 min;

Cook time: 4 min

Serving Size: 1;

Serves: 4;

Calories: 425g

Total Fat: 25g;

Protein: 44g;

Total Carbs: 10g

Dietary Fiber: 9g;

Sugar: 2g;

Sodium: 186mg

Ingredients

- 1 cup pepper jack cheese, hand-shredded
- 8 tortillas Tortilla Factory Low Carb Whole Wheat Tortillas
- 8 oz. cooked and shredded Chicken Breast
- 1 chopped and Roasted Bell Pepper
- T Cilantro
- 2 T Butter
- 1 cup plain Greek yogurt

Directions

Place ½ pat of butter in a skillet

Mix all the ingredients in a bowl except the yogurt

Place meat ingredients inside tortillas

Toast each side

Cut into 4 wedges

Top with yogurt and salsa, if desired

Freezing Instructions

Freeze in zip-lock bags. Place the yogurt in the fridge. Heat one minute in the microwave to thaw.

6   Chili Mac

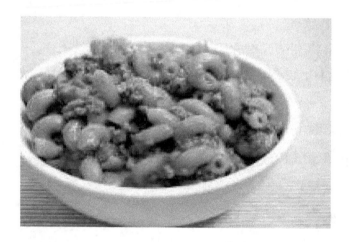

Prep time: 9 min;

Cook time: 9 min

Serving Size: 1/4;

Serves: 4;

Calories: 480

Total Fat: 24g;

Protein: 36g;

Total Carbs: 25g

Dietary Fiber: 6g;

Sugar: 4g;

Sodium: 995mg

Ingredients

- 1 lb ground Sirloin
- 1 chopped Onion
- 1 Chili Seasoning Mix, packet
- 1 cup tomato sauce
- 1 small can of Chunky Diced Tomatoes & Green Chilies
- 1 cup hand-shredded sharp cheddar
- 1 packet Splenda
- ½ cup Barilla Protein plus Elbow macaroni

Directions

Boil Barilla Protein plus Elbow macaroni until done, drain.

Brown the sirloin and onions in a large skillet.

Add the pasta, tomato sauce, diced tomatoes and green chilies, and chili seasoning mix.

Taste to see if you need to add water.

Serve in 4 bowls, topping each bowl with the cheddar cheese.

Freezer Directions

Place in four containers with lids, freeze. Microwave 2 minutes to thaw.

7   Cobb Salad

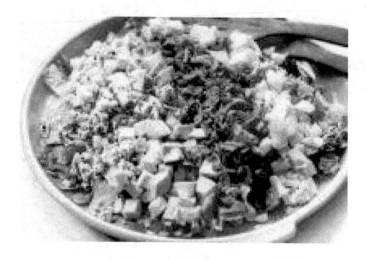

Prep time: 9 min;

Cook time: 9 min

Serving Size: 1;

Serves: 1;

Calories: 561

Total Fat: 34g;

Protein: 51g;

Total Carbs: 3.9g

Dietary Fiber: 6g;

Sugar: 1g;

Sodium: 802mg

Ingredients

- 1 slice Bacon or 1 T real bacon bits
- 1 grilled Chicken Breast, which has been cut into thin strips
- 1 cup Spring Mix Salad
- 1/2 cup grape tomatoes, sliced in half
- ½ avocado, sliced into small moons
- ¼ c pepper jack cheese, hand-shredded
- T Ken's Buttermilk Ranch Dressing

Directions

Assemble ingredients by sections.

Cover the entire bottom of the plate with lettuce.

In one corner (relative if you have a round plate) place the tomatoes.

In the opposite section place the avocado strips in a fan shape.

In the third section place the bacon bits.

In the fourth section place the hand-shredded cheese. In the center place the chicken.

Drizzle with the salad dressing and serve.

Freezing Instructions

The chicken can be frozen in a zip-lock bag. Microwave 1 minute to serve. The salad can be combined in one bowl, or packed in individual containers and placed in the fridge.

8   Cream of Mushroom Soup

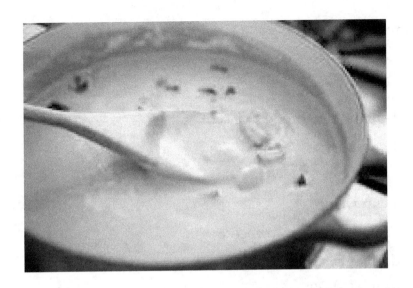

Prep time: 6 min;

Cook time: 4 min

Serving Size: 1 cup;

Serves: 4;

Calories: 210

Total Fat: 17g;

Protein: 10g;

Total Carbs: 3g

Dietary Fiber: 0.5g;

Sugar: 0g;

Sodium: 370mg

Ingredients

- 1-pound mushrooms, sliced
- 1 T butter
- ¼ cup cream
- 1 cup water
- ¼ grated Parmesan cheese
- dash of basil
- dash of black pepper

Directions

Microwave the mushrooms in the water for 4 minutes. Taste for the desired doneness.

Drain the mushrooms.

Place in blender with butter and cream and Parmesan.

Blend until creamy.

Pour into bowl and serve

Freezing Instructions

Freeze cooked soup in one cup containers. Microwave one minute, stir, and microwave one more minute to serve.

9 Cucumber Soup

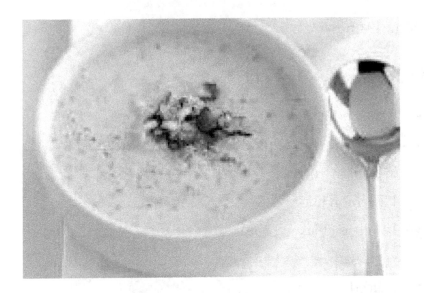

Prep time: 14 min;

Cook time: none

Serving Size: 1 cup;

Serves: 4;

Calories: 169

Total Fat: 12g;

Protein: 4g;

Total Carbs: 9g

Dietary Fiber: 5g;

Sugar: 6g;

Sodium: 494mg

Ingredients

- T minced garlic
- c English cucumbers, peeled and diced
- ½ c onion, diced
- 1 T lemon juice
- 1 ½ cups chicken broth
- ½ tsp salt
- 1 diced avocado
- ¼ tsp red pepper flakes
- ¼ cup diced parsley
- ½ cup Greek yogurt, plain

Directions

Place all the ingredients and emulsify by blending, except ½ c chopped cucumber.

Blend until smooth.

Pour into 4 servings.

Top with reserved cucumber.

Freezing Instructions

Freeze in one cup containers with lids. Let thaw to serve or microwave 2 minutes to serve hot.

10 Feta Cucumber Salad

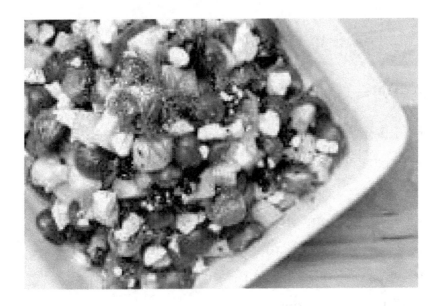

Prep time: 14 min;

Cook time: none

Serving Size: 1;

Serves: 4;

Calories: 142

Total Fat: 10g;

Protein: 4g;

Total Carbs: 7g

Dietary Fiber: 3g;

Sugar: 0g;

Sodium: 144mg

Ingredients

- 1 head of leaf lettuce, coarsely chopped
- 1 c baby spinach, trimmed, coarsely chopped
- ½ c diced red onion
- 1 c grape tomatoes, sliced in half
- ¼ c Feta cheese, crumbled
- cups plain Greek yogurt
- 2 T garlic powder
- 1 T dill
- 2 T lemon juice
- 2 English cucumbers, chopped with peels on
- 2 T olive oil
- ¼ tsp black pepper
- 1 small can black olives, sliced and drained (2.25 oz. can)
- ½ tsp mint or 3 mint leaves

Directions

Combine Greek yogurt, dill, garlic powder, mint, lemon juice, olive oil, ½ cup diced cucumber, and black pepper and emulsify by blending.

Taste and add salt. Add water by tablespoons if too thick.

Arrange on 4 plates the lettuce and spinach, tomatoes, cucumbers, and black olives.

Pour the dressing over the salad.

Top with the feta cheese.

Prep Directions

Mix the salad dressing and place in fridge in closed containers. Mix the salad and bag or place in covered containers in the fridge.

Place the feta cheese in a zip-lock bag in the fridge.

11 Seven Layer Salad

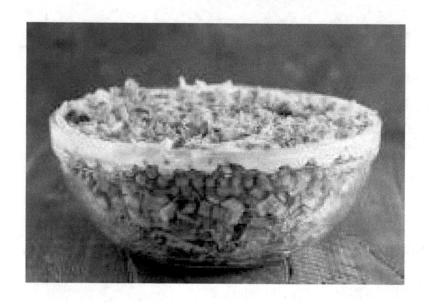

Prep time: 14 min;

Cook time: 9 min

Serving Size: 1;

Serves: 10;

Calories: 136

Total Fat: 7g;

Protein: 2g;

Total Carbs: 9g

Dietary Fiber: 2g;

Sugar: 0g;

Sodium: 324mg

Ingredients

- cups shredded butter lettuce
- cups shredded romaine lettuce
- 1 cup peas
- 1 cup diced bell peppers, red and yellow
- 1 cup grape tomatoes, halved
- 1 cup sliced celery
- ½ cup red onion
- ¾ cup Greek yogurt
- ¾ cup mayonnaise
- hard-boiled eggs
- 2 teaspoons cider vinegar
- 1 packet Splenda
- ¼ teaspoon garlic salt
- ½ cup pepper-jack cheese, hand-shredded
- 3 strips cooked bacon, crumbled

Directions

Using a large glass pan, 9x13 sized, layer the two lettuces.

Layer the peas, then the peppers, then the tomatoes, celery and onion.

Place the diced eggs next.

Combine the dressing ingredients: yogurt, mayonnaise, vinegar, garlic salt, Splenda, and a dash of black pepper.

Spread the dressing over the salad.

Garnish with the pepper-jack cheese and bacon.

Storage Instructions

Place in one cup containers. Close with a lid and refrigerate.

12 Shrimp and Cucumber Salad

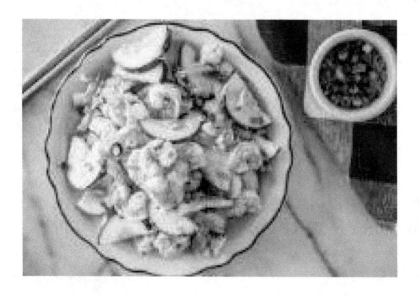

Prep time: 4 min;

Cook time: 0 min

Serving Size: 1/4;

Serves: 4;

Calories: 26g

Total Fat: 0g;

Protein: 2g;

Total Carbs: 3g

Dietary Fiber: 2g;

Sugar: 2g;

Sodium: 157mg

Ingredients

- English cucumbers
- 1/4 cup of red wine vinegar
- 2 tsp of Splenda
- 1/4 tsp salt
- ½ cup cooked shrimp

Directions

Peel the cucumbers so that they have stripes down the side.

Slice the cucumbers as thin as you can.

Mix the dressing of sugar, salt, and vinegar very well

Place thef cucumbers on a plate

Place the shrimp on top

Add the dressing and serve.

Prep Directions

Create the entire salad and place in a covered container in the fridge. Will keep 2 days.

13 Spinach Stuffed Portobello Mushrooms

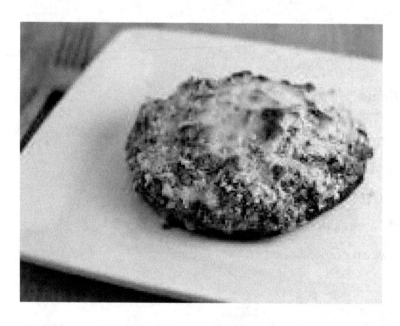

Prep time: 19 min;

Cook time: 28 min

Serving Size: 1;

Serves: 4;

Calories: 373

Total Fat: 28g;

Protein: 23g;

Total Carbs: 7g

Dietary Fiber: 1g;

Sugar: 2g;

Sodium: 681mg

Ingredients

- Portobello mushroom tops
- salt / pepper amount to taste
- 1 cup of ricotta cheese
- 1 cup chopped baby spinach
- ½ cup Parmesan cheese, hand-shredded
- 1 small can chopped or sliced black olives (2.25 oz.)
- ½ cup chunky vegetable marinara sauce
- ¼ cup mozzarella cheese, finely hand-shredded

Directions

Set the oven to 450F.

Line a 9 x 13-inch baking pan with some parchment paper.

Place the mushrooms smooth side against the parchment paper.

salt / pepper

Cook for about 24 minutes. Then remove it from heat source and pour off the liquid.

Mix the remaining ingredients except for the mozzarella cheese. Stuff into the tops of the mushrooms.

Bake 9 min.

Remove from heat source and sprinkle the top with the hand-shredded mozzarella.

Broil until the cheese is golden and melted. Serve.

Freezing Instructions

Freeze in individual zip-lock bags. Microwave for 2 minutes to serve.

14 Tuna Croquettes

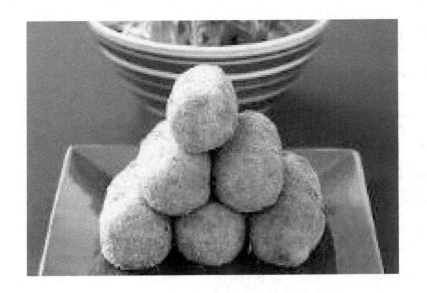

Prep time: 4 min;

Cook time: 9 min

Serving Size: 1 patty;

Serves: 4;

Calories: 105g

Total Fat: 5g;

Protein: 14g;

Dietary Fiber: 1g;

Total Carbs: 2g

Sugar: 0;

Sodium: 265mg

Ingredients

- 1 can tuna, drained
- 1 large egg
- 8 T grated Parmesan cheese
- T flax meal dash salt dash pepper
- 1 T minced onion

Directions

Blend all ingredients except the flax meal

Form into patties (¼ cup ea.)

Dip both sides in the flax meal

Fry until browned on both sides

Freezing Instructions

Place patties in one zip-lock bag each. Microwave 1 minute to serve.

15 Turkey Wraps

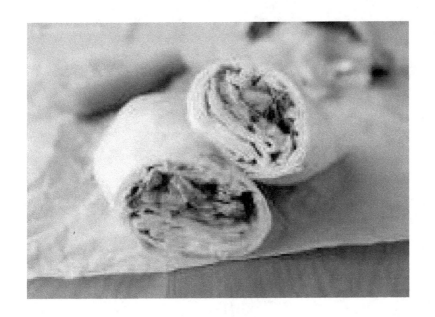

Prep time: 1 min;

Cook time: none

Serving Size: 1;

Serves: 1;

Calories: 154

Total Fat: 9g;

Protein: 12g;

Dietary Fiber: 0g;

Total Carbs: 2g

Sugar: 0g;

Sodium: 250mg

Ingredients

- slices deli turkey
- 1 oz. provolone cheese, sliced
- 1 lettuce leaf
- 1 tsp spicy brown mustard

Directions

Place turkey on the lettuce leaf

Spread with brown mustard

Top with the Provolone cheese

Roll into a burrito shape

Eat and enjoy!

Prep Instructions

Roll and prepare the wraps. Place on a paper towel. Place inside a zip-lock bag. Refrigerate until served.

Dinner

1   Easy Baked Chicken

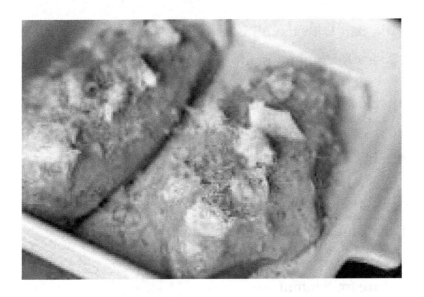

Preparation time: 10 minutes

Cooking time: 20 minutes

Servings: 4

Ingredients:

- bacon strips
- chicken breasts
- green onions, chopped
- ounces ranch dressing

- 1-ounce coconut aminos
- tablespoons coconut oil
- ounces cheddar cheese, grated

Directions:

Heat up a pan with the oil over high heat, add the chicken breasts, cook for 7 minutes, flip, and cook for 7 more minutes.

Heat up another pan over medium-high heat, add the bacon, cook until crispy, transfer to paper towels, drain the grease, and crumble.

Transfer the chicken breast to a baking dish, add the coconut aminos, crumbled bacon, cheese, and green onions on top, introduce in an oven, set on broiler, and cook at a high temperature for 5 minutes.

Divide on plates and serve.

2   Lemon Chicken

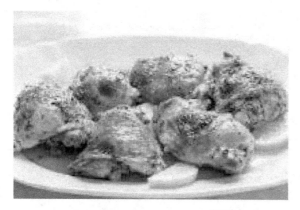

Preparation time: 10 minutes

Cooking time: 45 minutes

Servings: 6

Ingredients:

- 1 whole chicken, cut into medium-sized pieces
- Salt and ground black pepper, to taste
- Juice from 2 lemons
- Zest from 2 lemons
- Lemon rinds from 2 lemons

Directions:

Put the chicken pieces in a baking dish, season with some salt and pepper, and drizzle lemon juice.

Toss to coat well, add the lemon zest, and lemon rinds, place in an oven at 375°F and bake for 45 minutes.

Discard the lemon rinds, divide the chicken onto plates, drizzle sauce from the baking dish over it, and serve.

3   Slow-roasted Beef

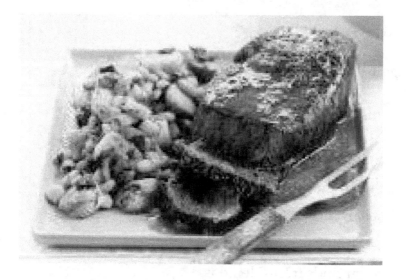

Preparation time: 10 minutes

Cooking time: 8 hours

Servings: 8

Ingredients:

- pounds beef roast
- Salt and ground black pepper, to taste
- ½ teaspoon celery salt
- teaspoons chili powder
- 1 tablespoon avocado oil
- 1 tablespoon sweet paprika
- A pinch of cayenne pepper
- ½ teaspoon garlic powder

- ½ cup beef stock
- 1 tablespoon garlic, minced
- ¼ teaspoon dry mustard

Directions:

Heat up a pan with the oil over medium-high heat, add the beef roast, and brown it on all sides.

In a bowl, mix the paprika with chili powder, celery salt, salt, pepper, cayenne, garlic powder, and dry mustard, and stir. Add the roast, rub well, and transfer it to a slow cooker.

Add the beef stock and garlic over roast, and cook on low for 8 hours.

Transfer the beef to a cutting board, leave it to cool, slice, and divide between plates.

Strain the juices from the pot, drizzle over the meat, and serve.

4 Salmon Meatballs

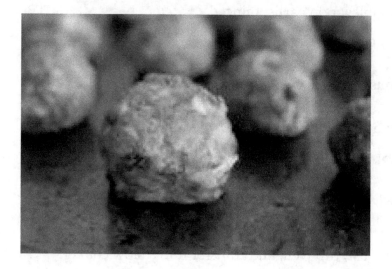

Preparation time: 10 minutes

Cooking time: 30 minutes

Servings: 4

Ingredients:

- tablespoons butter
- garlic cloves, peeled and minced
- ⅓ cup onion, peeled and chopped
- 1-pound wild salmon, boneless and minced
- ¼ cup fresh chives, chopped
- 1 egg
- tablespoons Dijon mustard
- 1 tablespoon coconut flour

- Salt and ground black pepper, to taste

For the sauce:

- garlic cloves, peeled and minced
- tablespoons butter
- tablespoons Dijon mustard
- Juice, and zest of 1 lemon
- cups coconut cream
- tablespoons fresh chives, chopped

Directions:

Heat up a pan with 2 tablespoons butter over medium heat, add the onion, and 2 garlic cloves, stir, cook for 3 minutes, and transfer to a bowl.

In another bowl, mix the onion and garlic with the salmon, chives, coconut flour, salt, pepper, 2 tablespoons mustard, and egg, and stir well.

Shape meatballs from the salmon mixture, place on a baking sheet, place in an oven at 350°F, and bake for 25 minutes.

Heat up a pan with 2 tablespoons butter over medium heat, add the 4 garlic cloves, stir, and cook for 1 minute.

Add the coconut cream, 2 tablespoons Dijon mustard, lemon juice, lemon zest, and chives, stir and cook for 3 minutes.

Take the salmon meatballs out of the oven, drop them into the Dijon sauce, toss, cook for 1 minute, and take off the heat.

Divide into bowls and serve.

5   Lemon and Garlic Pork

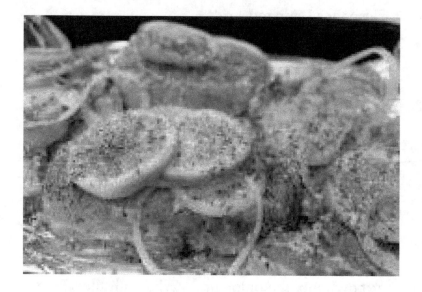

Preparation time: 10 minutes

Cooking time: 30 minutes

Servings: 4

Ingredients:

- tablespoons butter
- pork steaks, bone-in
- 1 cup chicken stock

- Salt and ground black pepper, to taste
- A pinch of lemon pepper
- tablespoons coconut oil
- garlic cloves, peeled and minced
- tablespoons fresh parsley, chopped
- 8 ounces mushrooms, chopped
- 1 lemon, sliced

Directions:

Heat up a pan with 2 tablespoons butter and 2 tablespoons oil over medium-high heat, add the pork steaks, season with salt and pepper, cook until they are brown on both sides, and transfer to a plate.

Return the pan to medium heat, add the rest of the butter, and oil, and half of the stock. Stir well, and cook for 1 minute.

Stir, and cook for 4 minutes after adding garlic and mushrooms.

Add the lemon slices, the rest of the stock, salt, pepper, and lemon pepper, stir and cook everything for 5 minutes.

Return the pork steaks to pan and cook everything for 10 minutes.

Divide the steaks and sauce between plates and serve.

Salad

1   Colorful Berry Salad

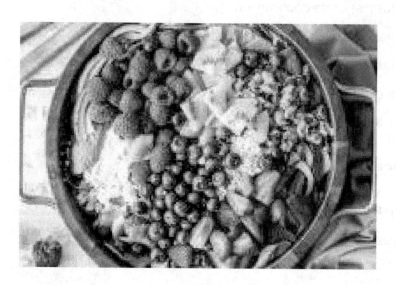

Ingredients:

- 1 cup Fresh Strawberries
- 1 cup Fresh Raspberries
- ¾ cup Fresh Blueberries
- ¾ cup Fresh Blackberries
- ¼ cup Fresh Cranberries
- 1 tablespoon Fresh Lime juice
- ½ tablespoon Pure Maple Syrup
- ¼ cup Almonds, toasted and chopped
- 1 tablespoon Mint Leaves, freshly chopped

Directions:

1 In a large serving bowl, mix all of the berries.

Add the lime juice and maple syrup and toss to coat. Garnish with the almonds and mint leaves before serving.

2 **Strawberry Spinach Salad**

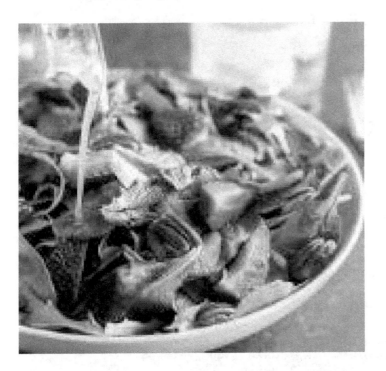

Ingredients:

For Vinaigrette:

- 1 small Garlic Clove, minced
- ¼ teaspoon Fresh Dill Weed
- ½ tablespoon Apple Cider Vinegar
- 1 tablespoon Fresh Lime juice

- 1 tablespoon Pure Maple Syrup
- Pinch of Freshly Ground Black Pepper

For Salad:

- 1 cup Fresh Strawberries, hulled and sliced
- cups Fresh Baby Spinach
- 1 Scallion, chopped
- 1 tablespoon Walnuts, chopped

Directions:

1   In a small bowl, mix the garlic, dill weed, vinegar, lime juice, maple syrup and black pepper.
2   In a large salad bowl, mix the strawberries, spinach, and scallion. Pour the vinaigrette over the salad and toss to coat well. Top with the walnuts and serve.
3   **Apple & Pear Salad**

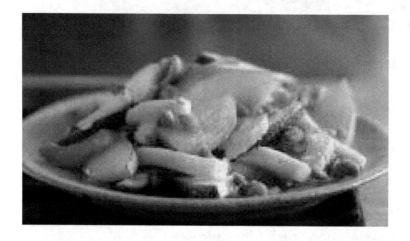

Ingredients:

- For Strawberry Vinaigrette:
- ½ cup Fresh Strawberries, hulled and sliced
- large Medjool Dates, pitted and chopped
- tablespoons Pecans, chopped
- ¼ cup Filtered Water
- ¼ cup Fresh Orange juice
- 1 tablespoon Apple Cider Vinegar

For Salad:

- 1 large Apple, peeled, cored and sliced
- 1 large Pear, peeled, cored and sliced
- cups Fresh Mixed Greens
- tablespoons Pumpkin Seeds, toasted

Directions:

1 In a blender, add all of the vinaigrette ingredients and pulse until smooth.
2 In a large salad bowl, mix the fruits and greens. Pour the vinaigrette over the salad and toss to coat well. Top with the pumpkin seeds and serve.

4   Mixed Citrus Salad

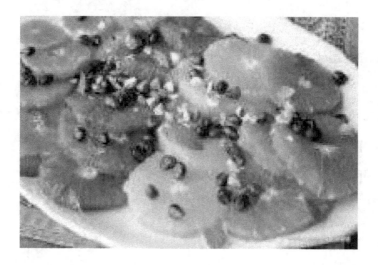

Ingredients:

- 1 Naval Orange, peeled, seeded and sectioned
- 1 Mandarin Orange, peeled, seeded and sectioned
- Grape Fruits, peeled, seeded and sectioned
- ½ tablespoon Pure Maple Syrup
- 1 tablespoon Mint Leaves, freshly chopped
- 1 teaspoon Orange Zest, freshly grated

Directions:

1   In a large serving bowl, mix all of the ingredients, except for the orange zest. Cover and refrigerate to chill before serving.
2   Garnish with the orange zest and serve.

Conclusion

I sincerely hope you are now equipped with a solid understanding of exactly what intermittent fasting is. Just as importantly, it is my wish that you are aware of the safe way for a woman to go about getting started with this lifestyle. There are a wide variety of methods that you can utilize on your fasting journey, the end goal is that all of them lead to the same destination: a healthier and happier you!

Remember that you are in control of your nutrition, health, and overall wellness. You do not have to follow intermittent fasting to achieve your goals, but this lifestyle is certainly a valuable tool to assist you with the health and physique you are striving for. Always remember that you are the one in control of what you eat and when you eat. If you choose to use intermittent fasting, that is a conscious choice that you are in complete control over. Never let any diet or exercise regimen gain control of you.

Intermittent fasting, although not a new idea by any means, has reemerged into the spotlight of the health and fitness industry and is now becoming the go-to nutrition plan for many people. If you sincerely commit to taking action and you try out this lifestyle for yourself, then it might just be the exact tool you needed to reach the health and weight goals that you desire. Now you have gained the understanding of how the female body works with intermittent fasting, and the knowledge of what to do, the choice is yours!

9 781914 033506